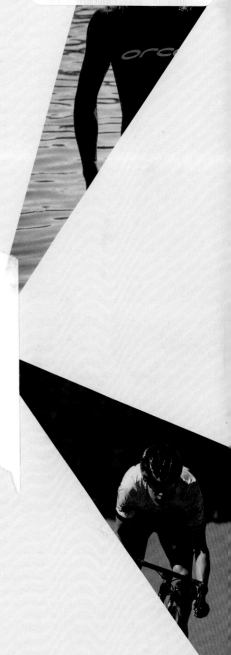

TRIATHLON

Published in 2018 by Dog 'n' Bone Books
An imprint of Ryland Peters & Small Ltd
20–21 Jockey's Fields   341 E 116th St
London WC1R 4BW   New York, NY 10029

www.rylandpeters.com

10 9 8 7 6 5 4 3 2 1

Text © Dominic Bliss 2018
Design © Dog 'n' Bone Books 2018

A CIP catalog record for this book is available from the Library of Congress and the British Library.

ISBN: 978 1 909313 96 5

Printed in China

Editor: Dawn Bates
Designer: Eoghan O'Brien
Photographer: Jason Bye
Additional photography credits: See below

Key: T=Top; B=Bottom; L=Left; R=Right; C=Center
p6 subman/Getty Images; p8 Caiaimage/Richard Johnson/Getty Images; p10 Ben Stansall/Staff/Getty Images; p12 Cultura/ Mickey Cashew/Getty Images; p13 (T) Kieferpix/Getty Images, (B) stefanschurr/Getty Images; p14 Kathy Cacicedo/Getty Images; p15 Gary Rohman/Getty Images; p16 subman/Getty Images; p18 pixdeluxe/Getty Images; p19 Caiaimage/Richard Johnson/ Getty Images; p21 Klaus Vedfelt/Getty Images; p22 Penny Wincer/Getty Images; p24 bluebeat76/Getty Images; p29 Koji Aoki/Getty Images; p30 Microgen/Getty Images; p35 Yasuyoshi Chiba/Staff/Getty Images; p36 Juice Images/Getty Images; p37 Mhaprang/Getty Images; p39 Microgen/Getty Images; p41 Squaredpixels/Getty Images; p42 Amriphoto/Getty Images; p45 Gary Newkirk/Staff/ Getty Images; p46 Hans Berggren/Getty Images; p55 Alex Caparros/Stringer/Getty Images; p61 Icon Sportswire/Contributor/Getty Images; p62 Stanislaw Pytel/Getty Images; p64 Johner Images/Getty Images; p65 Josef/Getty Images; p66 AGF/Contributor/ Getty Images; p67 pixdeluxe/Getty Images; p68 John B. Carnett/Contributor/Getty Images; p70 Johner Images/Getty Images; p71 Fabrice Coffrini/Staff/Getty Images; p72 Luca Sage/Getty Images; p75 Maridav/Getty Images; p79 Matthew Leete/Getty Images; p80 Charlie Crowhurst/Stringer/Getty Images; p81 Jordan Siemans/Getty Images; p83 Monkeybusinessimages/Getty Images; p84 Robert Daly/Getty Images; p92 Caiaimage/Richard Johnson/Getty Images; p93 Jacoblund/Getty Images; p110 Thomas Barwick/Getty Images; p112 Yann Coatsaliou/Contributor/Getty Images; p114 Alexander Hassenstein/Staff/Getty Images; p115 Mike Powell/Staff/Getty Images; p118 Gary Newkirk/Staff/Getty Images; p119 Thomas Barwick/Getty Images; p120 (T) 7000/ Getty Images; p126 Tim Williams/Contributor/Getty Images; p129 Leon Neal/Stringer/Getty Images; p130 Leon Neal/Staff/Getty Images; p131 Adam Pretty/Getty; p132 Ezra Shaw/Staff/Getty Images; p134–135 Jan Hetfleisch/Stringer/Getty Images; p136 Ezra Shaw/Staff/Getty Images; p137 Icon Sports Wire/Contributor/Getty Images; p138 Kai-Otto Melau/Contributor/Getty Images; p139 Neil Kerr/Stringer/Getty Images; p140 Jack Taylor/Stringer/Getty Images; p142 Icon Sportswire/Contributor/Getty Images

ACKNOWLEDGMENTS

Many experts helped with the writing of this book. Thank you to all of them.

Main triathlon consultant: Ian Rooke, triathlon coach and triathlon retail expert from Sigma Sport.

Swimming consultant: Paul Newsome, head coach at swimming coaching company Swim Smooth [swimsmooth.com].

Triathlon training consultant: Simon Ward, from The Triathlon Coach [thetriathloncoach.com].

Technical bike consultant: Ebba Merrington, director of Velo City Cycling, a London-based mobile bike repair service [ww.velocitycycling.co.uk].

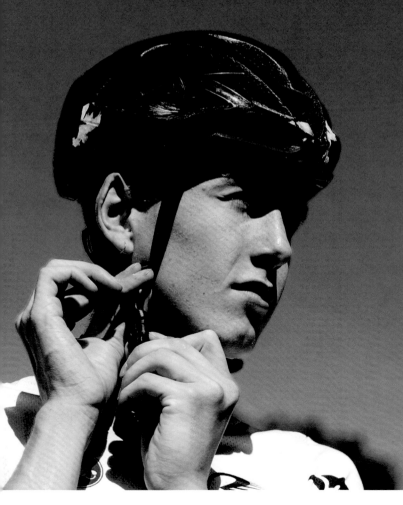

Dominic Bliss

TRIATHLON

Expert training and race advice
for beginners and improvers

DOG 'n' BONE

Contents

Introduction   6

Chapter
01
THE BASICS 10

Chapter
02
SWIM TRAINING   26

Chapter
03
BIKE TRAINING   46

Chapter
04
RUN TRAINING   72

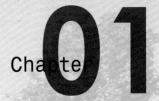

Chapter 05

TRANSITION TRAINING   84

Chapter 06

TRAINING SCHEDULES   90

Chapter 07

RACE DAY   110

Chapter 08

THE WORLD'S GREATEST TRIATHLONS   132

Index   144

INTRODUCTION

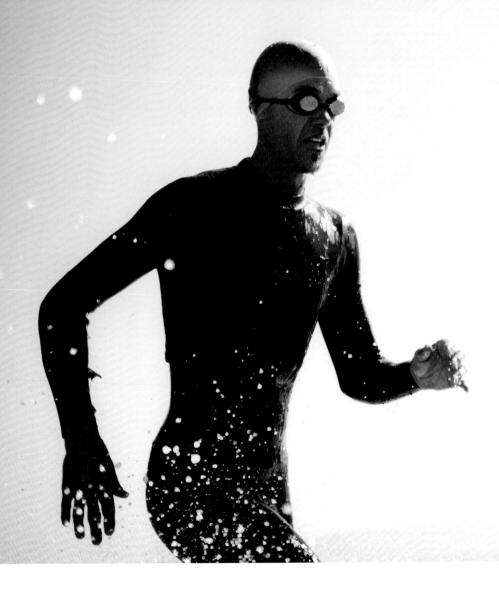

So you want to be a triathlete? Well, you're certainly not alone. According to the latest figures from the International Triathlon Union, there are over 3.5 million people regularly competing in triathlons around the world, and more than 9,000 official triathlon clubs.

That's quite a staggering number—and even more impressive when you consider that the sport is only around 40 years old.

Although swim—bike—run races had been held in various primitive forms ever since the bicycle was invented in the 1800s, it wasn't until 1974 that the term "triathlon" was first used. The venue was Mission Bay, a huge saltwater lagoon in San Diego, California, and the organizers were Jack Johnstone and his colleagues from the San Diego Track Club. They called it the Mission Bay Triathlon. "When we were ordering the award trophies, the shop owner asked me how to spell "triathlon," Johnstone recalls of that historic September day. "He hadn't found it in any dictionary."

A rather modest field of 46 participants (they weren't known as triathletes in those days) turned up after work to compete across 6 miles (10km) of running, 5 miles (8km) of cycling, and 500 yards (500m) of swimming.

For the bike section, many were astride beach cruisers and three-speed leisure bikes. "Most didn't own racing bikes and some were marginal swimmers at best," Johnstone remembers. "Yet they had the adventuresome spirit to come out after a day of work to participate in a new athletic event."

So the triathlon was born.

IRONMAN

Four years later, in 1978, in Hawaii, one of those original Mission Bay triathletes, John Collins, found himself embroiled in a heated debate with fellow sportsmen about whether it was swimmers, runners, or cyclists who were the fittest. To settle the argument once and for all, they decided to stage the first ever Ironman triathlon, incorporating three local endurance races—the 2.4-mile (4-km) Waikiki rough water swim, the 112-mile (180km) around Oahu bike race, and the 26.2-mile (42-km) Honolulu Marathon. There were 15 entrants, 12 finishers, and the winner was Gordon Haller, with a time of 11 hours, 46 minutes, and 58 seconds. (It's interesting to compare that to the current top Ironman competitors, who regularly post winning times of around 8 hours.)

AN OLYMPIC EVENT

The idea of combining three such basic sports into one race quickly sparked the imagination of sports event organizers. By the late 1980s, there were regular triathlons in countries all across the globe. The International Triathlon Union was founded in 1989, with its chief aim being gaining Olympic status for the sport.

It was at the Sydney Olympics in 2000 that triathlon made its debut.

Nowadays, every week of the year, there are hundreds, if not thousands, of triathlons staged worldwide. How proud those original Mission Bay triathletes must feel, especially those who had competed on the three-speed leisure bikes.

A POPULAR SPORT

So just how has this unorthodox combination of swimming, biking, and running so rapidly cemented itself as a global leisure pursuit? Why is triathlon so amazingly popular?

Fitness and weight loss are, of course, major factors. Many triathletes are office employees, chained to a desk all day, but keen to stave off the middle-aged spread once they are released from work. Charity is an incentive, too, with many competitors raising money for good causes. Unlike some sports, triathlon is surprisingly easy to train for: all three disciplines can be honed in a gym that has a pool. Running or cycling training can even be done as part of the commute to work.

But there are perhaps more atavistic reasons for why we want to subject ourselves to this

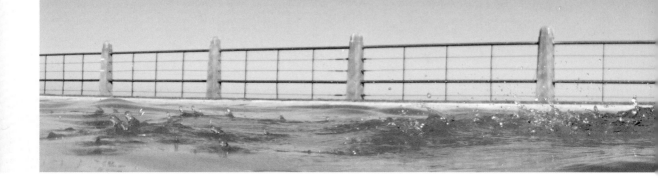

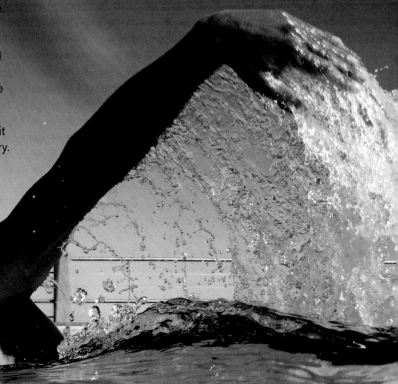

multisport endurance test. In the developed world, at least, we are mollycoddled, with sedentary jobs and comfortable homes. We no longer hunt for our food or battle with neighboring tribes. For several generations, most of us have avoided military conscription. So, come the weekend, we're searching for adventure, and what better way to find it than swimming across a lake before clocking up miles on a bike and then in our running shoes.

HOW TO USE THIS BOOK

If you're a triathlon virgin, you will find this book invaluable, since it tells you everything you need to compete in—and hopefully enjoy— your first race. Or maybe you've competed in a triathlon before, and need some pointers on how to improve or make it a more positive experience. Perhaps you're fairly fit already, just not in triathlon. Maybe you've done a handful of 5k races, or some charity bike rides, and you feel you need a new challenge that's a bit more competitive. If so, triathlon is the perfect place to take your next step up.

Don't assume that you need to be fit to benefit from the advice in this book. Quite the contrary. Even if you're a bit of a couch potato, there's plenty here to inspire you both mentally and physically to get race-ready. If you need a boost, you've come to the right place.

Whatever level you're starting at, you'll find it useful to read Chapter 1 first, as it gives you some basic pointers on training, equipment, nutrition, and motivation. Then there are separate chapters for each discipline. You may want to start by reading up on the area you feel is your weakest—for many beginners, it's swimming. Chapter 5 talks you through the important transition stages which, if executed well, can improve your finishing times. There are training schedules in Chapter 6—use these as a guideline only and adapt them as necessary, depending on your other commitments and the areas you most need to improve. Chapter 7 talks you through race day and how to make it a positive experience and avoid the pitfalls.

CHAPTER 1

THE BASICS

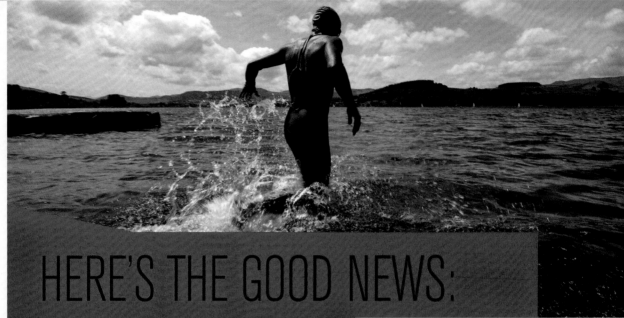

HERE'S THE GOOD NEWS:

Your first few triathlons won't be as difficult as you think. If you're reading this book, it's likely you're planning to do the two shortest distances, either a Sprint or Olympic triathlon, and that means your mission isn't enormously demanding. This is not some false psychology designed to trick you into being confident. It's the truth. A Sprint-distance triathlon—the distance that most beginners start with—requires you to swim 750m, cycle 20km, and run 5km. With some decent training, these distances are easily achievable, even if you're starting out relatively unfit.

THE RACE DISTANCES

All official triathlons are in this order: swim, bike, run. There are four commonly staged distances:

≡ **SPRINT**: 750-m (820-yard) swim, 20-km (12-mile) bike, 5-km (3-mile) run

≡ **OLYMPIC** (or standard): 1.5-km (0.9-mile) swim, 40-km (25-mile) bike, 10-km (6-mile) run)

≡ **HALF IRONMAN** (or Ironman 70.3): 1.9-km (1.2-mile) swim, 90-km (56-mile) bike, 21.1-km (13-mile) run (a half marathon)

≡ **IRONMAN** 3.8-km (2.4-mile) swim, 180-km (112-mile) bike, 42.2-km (26.2-mile) run (a marathon)

NOTE: For simplicity, the book uses metric distances, which aligns with International Triathlon Union competition rules.

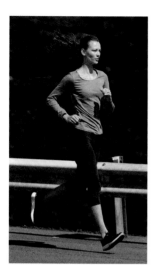

And don't forget, you won't be alone. At this level, there will be loads of other triathlon virgins, or "newbies," as they're known, taking part, feeling just as nervous as you are. Don't forget, you're not going for any records. In order to hold your head high, all you need to do is cross the finish line to say you've completed a triathlon. Don't feel daunted. It's really not that tricky, unless, for some bizarre reason you've signed up for an Ironman event as a race virgin. In which case you're obviously so hard-core, that nothing's going to put you off!

Don't, however, underestimate the need to do the basic training. If you try to complete your first triathlon without doing any training, you'll risk injury, and undergo a lot of suffering as you struggle through the distances. There's no getting round it: training takes time and effort. You've probably got a full-time job and you may have family commitments. Trying to fit a swim, bike, or run into your already busy schedule is going to require serious organization, but it will all be well worth it.

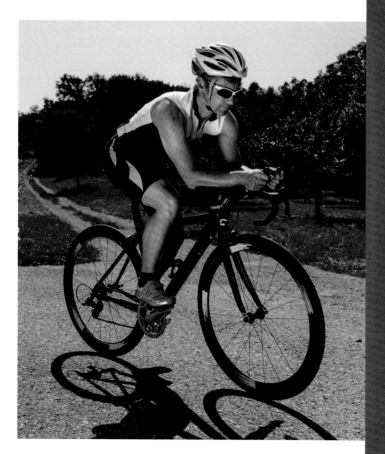

Triathlons are normally split into five sections:

≡ The swim section

≡ T1 [transition]—the time you spend in the transition area between the swim and the bike ride

≡ The bike section

≡ T2 [transition]—the time you spend in the transition area between the bike ride and the run

≡ The run section to the finish line

You may be a virgin triathlete, but that doesn't mean you have to make your first race a Sprint distance. You can happily debut with an Olympic triathlon. It all depends on your base level of fitness in the three disciplines. If you class yourself as extremely unfit, it's wise to opt for the Sprint distance first time round.

THE EQUIPMENT

Experienced triathletes will have more gear than you think is humanly possible: a specialist tri bike with tri bars/aero bars, perhaps an aero helmet, cycling shoes and clipless pedals, a tri suit…

Don't be intimidated. As a beginner, you can get away with a limited amount of equipment that won't cost you the earth.

Later on, if you discover you love the sport, you can upgrade your gear as you improve.

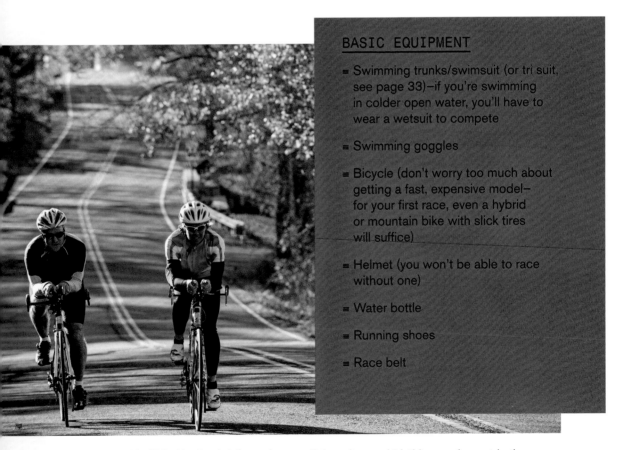

BASIC EQUIPMENT

≡ Swimming trunks/swimsuit (or tri suit, see page 33)—if you're swimming in colder open water, you'll have to wear a wetsuit to compete

≡ Swimming goggles

≡ Bicycle (don't worry too much about getting a fast, expensive model—for your first race, even a hybrid or mountain bike with slick tires will suffice)

≡ Helmet (you won't be able to race without one)

≡ Water bottle

≡ Running shoes

≡ Race belt

You'll find in-depth information on all the advanced triathlon equipment in the training sections on swimming, biking, and running, in Chapters 2–4.

TRAINING

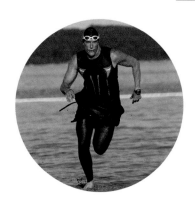

When you sign up for your first triathlon, give yourself a minimum of three months to train. That's plenty of time to get race-ready, even if, right now, you're unfit and very busy with work and family. As with any sport, if your body's not used to the activity, start out gently and build up slowly. Don't risk injuring yourself in the first week by jumping straight in at the deep end. (See Chapter 6: Training Schedules, pages 90–109.)

Once you've signed up and paid your race entry fee, you'll notice an immediate psychological switch—there's nothing like a race date to focus the mind. Use that focus to make a start on your training.

Many triathlon debutants struggle to find the time they need to train (unless they're students or unemployed, in which case they should don Lycra the minute they get out of bed). Yes, you've got three disciplines to train for, but the good news is that two of them, at least, are reasonably easy to shoehorn into your daily schedule. Busy job? Is it possible to commute to work by bike,

or run part of the distance? Burdened down by childcare? Get yourself a baby buggy you can run with and put a child seat on the back of your bike. Or if your kids are older, they can ride their bikes with you while you run round the park alongside them.

One of the reasons triathlon has become such a popular sport is because all three disciplines can be practiced at the gym on the stationary bike and treadmill and by using the pool, if there is one. Try to hit the gym at lunchtime or before/after work whenever possible.

Two at a time
Jonathan Brownlee, triathlon champion

"It's really impractical to do all three disciplines in one session, especially when it's cold. Train to be as good as you can be at all three individually and then put it all together on race day."

Balancing the disciplines

Training for triathlon is like trying to maintain relationships with three different lovers. Each discipline clamors for your attention. You inevitably prefer one to the other two. One of them makes you feel quite anxious. You'd love to combine all three, but you're not quite sure how that's going to work.

Remember that you don't have to give all three triathlon disciplines equal attention. Sometimes you need to spend more time on your weaker sport. You'll quickly figure out which is your weakest discipline (and for most beginners this is the swim). If you need to compensate, spend more time in the pool or on the bike during training, but don't neglect your strongest disciplines.

Many triathletes combine two disciplines during training, maybe linking a swim with a bike ride, or a bike ride with a run (this is called a brick—see pages 87 and 88), but hardly anyone combines all three.

Transition training

Seasoned triathletes will remind you that their sport has four disciplines, not just three. They consider transitions— the changeover from the swim to the bike, then the bike to the run—a whole discipline of its own. And quite rightly, given that it's an area where so much time can be lost or gained. It's important to practice transitions: quick wetsuit removal (see page 121); rapid mounting and dismounting of the bike (see pages 124 and 127); helmet straps and shoe laces (see page 128)… these are crucial. (See Chapter 5: Transition Training.)

Don't overtrain

Many athletes, both amateur and professional, are guilty of overtraining. Determined to post great results in a race, they push themselves to complete more exercise than their bodies can tolerate. In extreme cases, it can actually end up reducing their fitness and make them susceptible to illness

Pro-Tip

Concentrate on your weakest discipline
Julie Whaley, Absolute Triathlon Coaching

"Perhaps you find you're overwhelmed by everything; by the enormity of your task. I try to rein my triathletes in a bit. I find they're like children in a sweet shop: they want to do all three disciplines every single day. That's not the way to look at it. If swimming isn't your strength, for example, and you're less comfortable with that, you should focus more on swimming training. That way, when it comes to the race, you'll feel a lot more comfortable with the swim section."

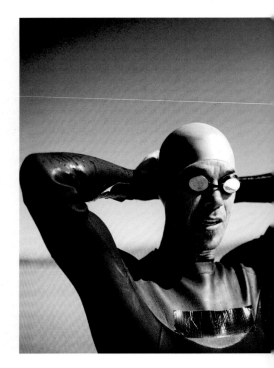

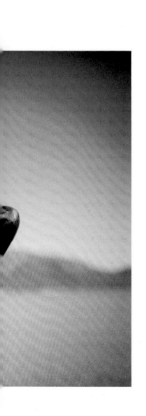

and infection. It's important to be aware of how your body feels. If you've really pushed yourself in training and you feel very fatigued, then give your body a rest. After training you might feel aches and pains in your body (known as delayed onset muscle soreness, or DOMS). Fail to let these recover and you risk injuring yourself. Within your training schedule, rest days are crucial (see pages 22 and 93). So respect them. If you do get injured, definitely rest and, if possible, see a physiotherapist. It will make all the difference to your recovery.

Train with other athletes

There's no better way to inject yourself with a bit of motivation than by training with other athletes. You could always join a triathlon club—most will welcome beginners, and you'll glean lots of valuable advice from seasoned triathletes. But if this sounds a bit too serious, then why not just ask your fit friends (or your other half) to accompany you on a training session? So many people regularly swim, bike, and run that you're sure to know someone who's more experienced than you in each of the three disciplines. They will give you that extra psychological boost you need to get out of the house and exercise.

Training journal

Keeping a record of your training will incentivize you. It doesn't have to be anything too technical, and should take you a couple of minutes to complete after each training session.

There are plenty of training apps available that allow you to log your progress and encourage you to push yourself physically, but an old-fashioned notebook will work just as well. It's a great idea to note down the sport you work on, the time you spend

on it, the distances you cover, and the intensity of your effort. The advantages of keeping a journal are:

≡ You'll feel a real sense of accomplishment, and you'll be able to monitor your progress.

≡ It will stop you accidentally neglecting one of the triathlon disciplines and allow you to spot any weaknesses.

≡ It will enable you to see what time of day you train most efficiently.

≡ It will help you work out how much food and drink you should ideally be consuming.

≡ It will help you discover which items of clothing and equipment work best, and which don't.

Note down:

≡ Swim, bike, or run?

≡ Time of day and distance covered

≡ Intensity (i.e. percentage of your maximum output)

≡ Food and drink you consumed before, during, and after training

≡ Any new clothing and equipment you were testing

≡ How you felt physically and psychologically during and after

Expert triathletes use heart rate monitors and, after training, often note down their average heart rate in their training journal, but at beginner level this isn't essential.

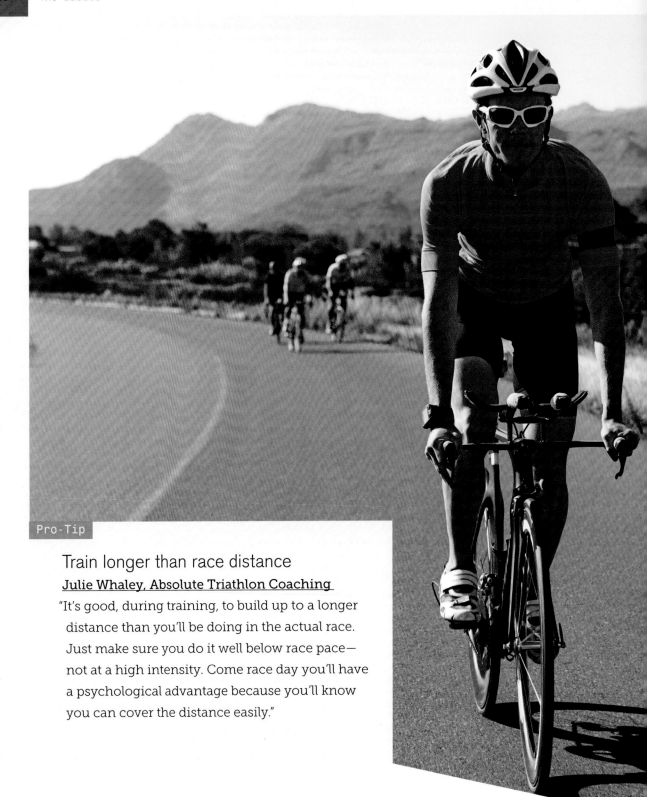

Pro-Tip

Train longer than race distance
<u>Julie Whaley, Absolute Triathlon Coaching</u>

"It's good, during training, to build up to a longer
distance than you'll be doing in the actual race.
Just make sure you do it well below race pace—
not at a high intensity. Come race day you'll have
a psychological advantage because you'll know
you can cover the distance easily."

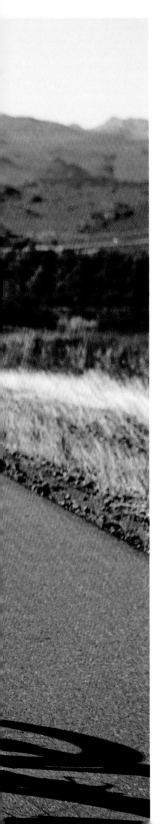

Tapering your training

As race day approaches, you should cut back on the intensity of your training, which is called tapering. The benefits are that it allows your muscles to heal and feel fresh on race day, and it lets your glycogen stores build up in the days leading up to the race.

Different triathletes taper by different amounts, depending on the length of the triathlon, their fitness, and their age. Experts don't agree exactly on how much you should taper. But, as a general rule, if you're doing a Sprint- or Olympic-distance triathlon, think about cutting down your training distances and intensity incrementally in the final two weeks. It doesn't mean you should stop training altogether, however.

The 12-week training schedules for Sprint and Olympic distances on pages 94–109 incorporate this tapering.

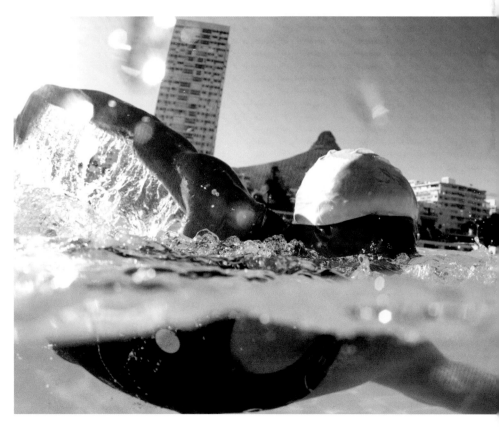

NUTRITION

A great diet makes for a great athlete. The food intake for triathlon is no different to that needed for any other endurance sport. There's no secret science to this, and at beginner-level triathlon you certainly don't need to be taking food supplements, but you should be eating a well-balanced, healthy diet. This should include:

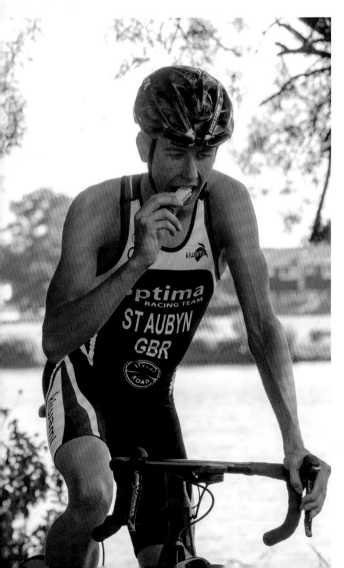

≡ A decent amount of carbohydrate. Carbs have earned a bad reputation in recent years, but there's no getting away from it: if you're planning a long training session, then you will need the energy that carbs provide. Aim for complex carbohydrates, such as wholegrain bread, pasta, and cereals, fruits, vegetables, nuts, seeds, and legumes. Go big on the fruits and vegetables since they have the added benefit of being great sources of vitamins and minerals, boosting your immune system and overall health.

≡ Lots of lean protein, such as chicken, turkey, fish, and eggs. (Vegetarians and vegans need to be more inventive to consume enough vegetable protein. Think beans, lentils, chickpeas, tofu, peanuts, and soya milk and yogurt.) Protein will help repair muscles that become damaged by lots of training.

≡ Small amounts of unsaturated fats, such as olive oil, unroasted nuts, seeds, avocado, oily fish, and peanut butter.

It's important not to train on an empty stomach, nor on a completely full stomach. You'll know what works best for you, but the general consensus is that you shouldn't eat a meal less than two hours before you start training. You will always need to eat as part of your recovery process after your training sessions. Unless you're doing a particularly long bike ride, it's unlikely you'll need to eat during training at this level.

Energy gels

Don't be fooled by the sports industry marketing people. As a beginner triathlete, you do not need to consume loads of energy gels. Many of them are packed full of simple sugars and will make your stomach feel very queasy. If you really want to eat during training, take fruit or cereal bars instead.

Hydration

There are plenty of post-exercise drinks (full of electrolytes) on the market. Don't obsess about these. Normal water does the job too. Make sure you drink plenty of water before, during, and after your training sessions, especially in hot weather. As you sweat, it's easy to dehydrate surprisingly quickly. This will slow you down and reduce the benefit of the training session in the first place.

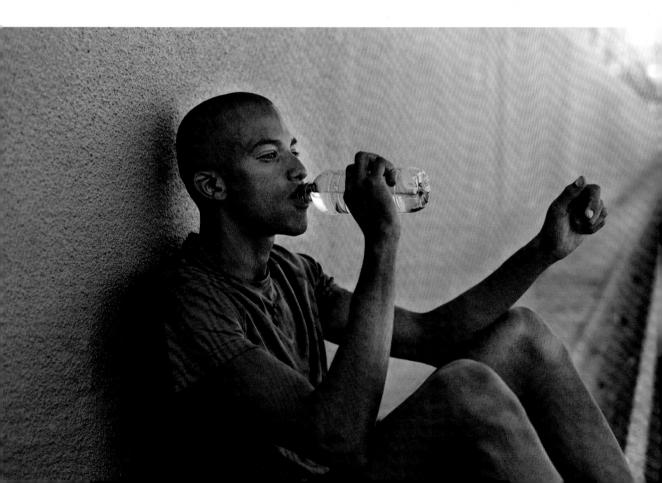

RECOVERY

How you treat your body when you're not exercising can be just as important as the actual training. That's why it's crucial to build rest days into your training schedule. Here are some other key ways to aid recovery.

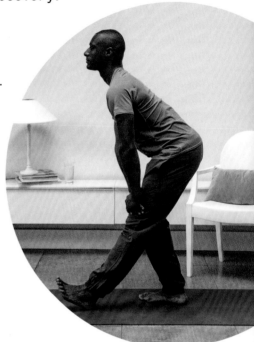

≡ Sleep: aim for around eight hours a night, if possible.

≡ Eat well and stay hydrated: see pages 20–21.

≡ Cooling down: just as important as warming up for exercise is cooling down. It will reduce muscle soreness and help flush out excess lactic acid.

≡ Massage: unfortunately, not all of us have access to a personal sports masseur. Ask your other half to help ease your sore muscles or self-massage if you have to, using a foam roller or even just an old tennis ball.

REALISTIC GOALS

When you're first starting out in triathlons, it's important that you are realistic about your goals. Don't imagine that you can transform yourself overnight from a 5-k runner to a triathlete—it's just not possible. Besides, you'll risk serious injury. You need to work up gradually to the longer distances, both physically and mentally, in swimming, biking, and running.

Before you even start training, decide whether your goal is simply to complete the triathlon, or to post an impressive time. Head coach Paul Newsome (see opposite) believes debutant triathletes should be completers rather than competers.

Competers and completers
Paul Newsome, head coach at Swim Smooth

"Triathletes are often split into two categories: those looking to compete
and those who just want to complete. Completers love setting themselves
a challenge, which feels a little scary but creates a real buzz of excitement
at the same time. They use that heady mix of fear and excitement
for motivation to train for the big day. They try to fit training and
racing in around their normal life and see their chosen sport as part
of a bigger picture.

"Competers, on the other hand, are all about performance. Just finishing
an event isn't enough; it's about where they place, and improving on
their previous performances. They train hard and can't help but get a little
obsessed about how things are going. Rather than fitting training around
their lives, they end up fitting life around their training.

"Unfortunately, competers often look down on completers, thinking, 'If you
just trained harder and believed in yourself a bit more, you could be so
much faster than you are.' That's undoubtedly true, but would getting
more focused ultimately make them happier?

"Completers are in fact very good at something that competers are very
bad at: letting themselves win. Completers set themselves a challenging
goal, but something that is actually achievable. And they feel great when
they reach that goal. Competers, on the other hand, tend to set their goals
just out of reach so that they rarely hit them. Or, when they do hit them,
they immediately move their targets higher again. Rather than taking
satisfaction from training hard and doing their best, they judge
themselves and their self-worth from their pure performance.
All too often things end in failure."

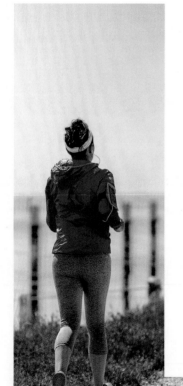

Goal-setting

<u>Midgie Thompson, mental performance and lifestyle coach</u>

"Have goals that are within your control, and that you can achieve. Sports psychologists often talk about the difference between outcome goals and performance goals, encouraging athletes to aim for the latter. In terms of endurance races, an outcome goal would be: 'I want to finish my triathlon in under two hours, placed in the top 100.' A performance goal would be: 'I want to remain confident throughout the race, I want to manage those race nerves to fuel my performance, and I want to make sure I cross the finish line, regardless of the time.'

"You don't always have control over the outcome goals. Outcomes can be influenced by other factors such as poor weather, stronger athletes, or getting a puncture in the bike section. All these could slow you down or place you right down the field. If you set yourself outcome goals and then don't achieve them, you will give yourself negative feedback and this may discourage you from continuing with the sport. Focus on those elements you can control: your attitude, your focus, your confidence. Remain positive, complete the race, enjoy yourself, enjoy the environment. If your goal is to cross the line, regardless of the time, then you will feel positive after the race. This gives you positive feedback and you're more likely to continue with the sport."

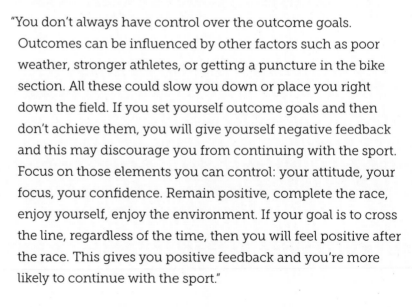

STAYING MOTIVATED

Everyone finds it much easier to train for triathlon in
the spring and summer months. It's warmer, it stays lighter
longer, and (usually) there's less mud on the ground. But if
your triathlon is taking place in the spring, you'll need
to get some good, long hours of training completed during
the latter stages of the winter. If you work a full-time job,
that means you'll either be training inside a gym, or you'll
be outside in the cold and the dark.

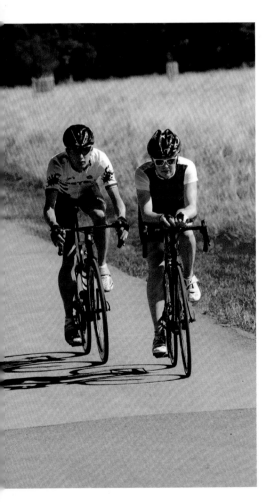

Building a run or bike ride into your commute to and from work is one great solution. But when it isn't possible, how do you motivate yourself to train once you get home and every part of you simply wants to curl up in front of the TV? One good tip is to change into your running or cycling clothing the minute you get home from work. That way you'll be less tempted to skip the exercise. Do lots of warm-up exercises inside your house so that your body is ready to perform before you head out of the door.

Music is a good motivation tool, too. If you're running or cycling off-road, it's normally safe to have headphones in your ears. There's nothing like an upbeat tune to get the blood pumping. Not only will it inspire you on cold, wet evenings, but it has actually been proven to increase endurance.

Training with a friend (or your partner) will further incentivize you. Even better if that friend plans to compete in the same triathlon. You'll find it very difficult to dodge a training session when your training partner is ringing at your doorbell, insisting you come for a ride or a run.

However motivated you are, though, there will always be times when you simply can't drag yourself out of the door. Pressures of work, family commitments, niggling injuries... these can all conspire to scupper your best intentions. Don't worry. This happens even to top professional triathletes. You can always make up for it by training slightly harder the following day.

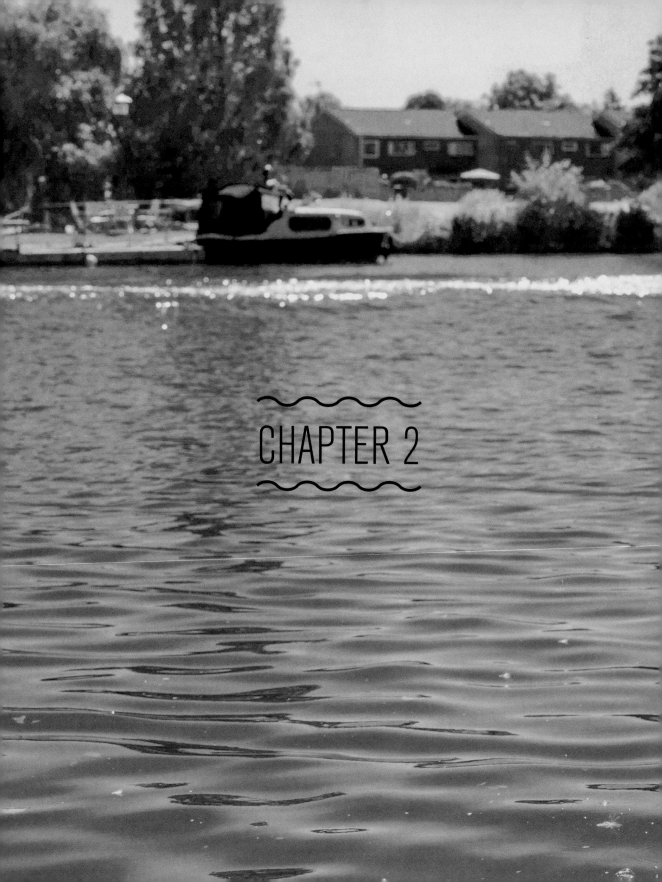

CHAPTER 2

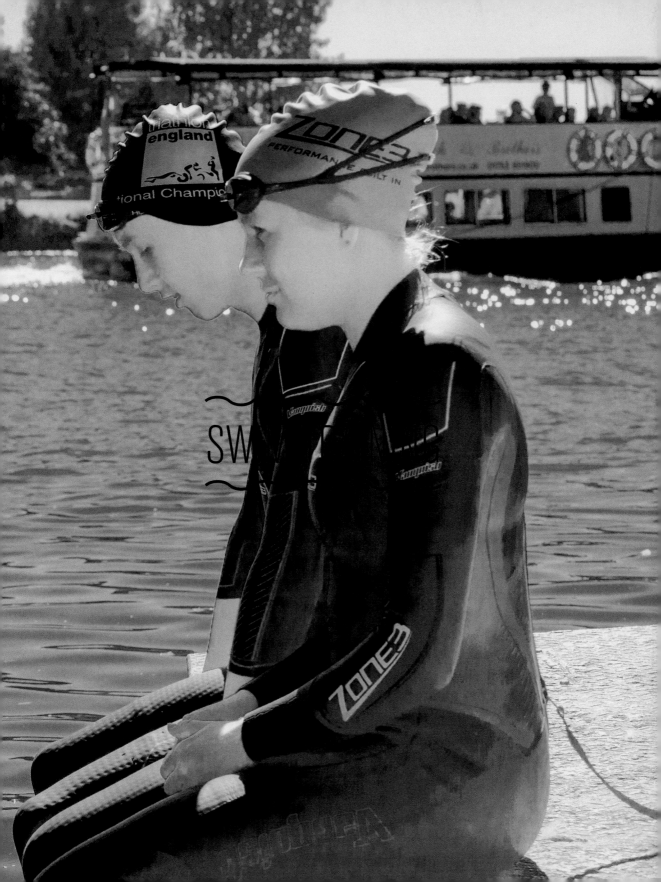

FOR SWIM TRAINING, YOU NEED ACCESS TO A SWIMMING POOL OR A NICE, WARM LAKE.

There's no getting round this. That's why debutant triathletes often find the swim training the hardest discipline of all three. After all, you can run and cycle pretty much anywhere, including inside a gym, but to swim, ideally you need water that is safe, flat, and warm. Some longer races will subject you to choppy, open water, in which case you'll need to emulate those conditions for some of your training, but entry-level triathlons normally place you in swimming pools or placid lakes. So step one of your swim training, before you even dip your toe in the water, is to locate your nearest pool or lake.

LOCAL SWIMMING POOL

Training at your local pool is likely to be your easiest and cheapest option. Unfortunately, it might also be the grubbiest, especially if it's a busy pool. Choose a pool that's close to home or your place of work so that you can't make excuses not to train. Find out when the pool is set up for lane swimming, and when it's least busy. For obvious reasons, before work, lunchtimes, and just after work are the busiest times, but during the day school lessons and groups of grannies can also halt your progress. Just before the pool closes in the evening can often be a quiet time. Print out the pool opening times and the lane schedules, and stick them to your refrigerator door or above your desk. Busy pools mean you'll need to be opportunistic about snatching training slots when you can.

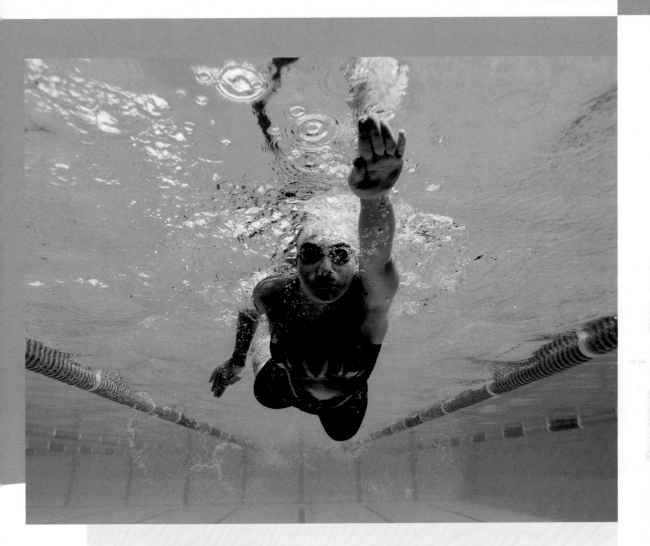

PRIVATE CLUBS

If you're lucky enough to be a member of a private club, you're likely to have access to a lovely swimming pool, which you might even get all to yourself sometimes. If there's a gym there, you can use the stationary bikes and the running treadmills to train for your other two disciplines.

It's worth considering joining a club for the duration of your training as, although it may put a strain on your wallet, it will allow you to train after dark and in all weathers. You may even bump into a few triathlon debutants like yourself or more experienced triathletes who can offer you invaluable advice.

OPEN WATER

If your chosen triathlon is being staged in open water then, sooner or later, you're going to need to train in the stuff. Unless you live in the tropics, this means you'll need a wetsuit (see opposite). Lakes and reservoirs are the best option since there are no currents or tides, and they're (normally) flat. Avoid swimming in canals, urban rivers, and stagnant lakes, and never swim in open water alone.

Swimming in the sea is another possibility although, depending on the current and tides, it can be dangerous. Opt for sheltered sections of sea and wear a brightly colored swimming hat so you are visible in the water. A clunk on the head from a jet ski will really ruin your day, not to mention your training schedule. Be aware that waves can cause seasickness and disorientation, even for experienced swimmers.

River swimming is an option, but you'll need to check with landowners whether access is allowed. Swim against rather than with the current and you'll find you get a much better workout. But it comes with a particular set of hazards—pollution, boats, driftwood, fishing tackle... all these can throw you off your stroke.

In fresh water, wear waterproof plasters over any cuts you might have. Don't jump straight in unless you're sure of what lurks beneath. For the same reason, consider wearing footwear.

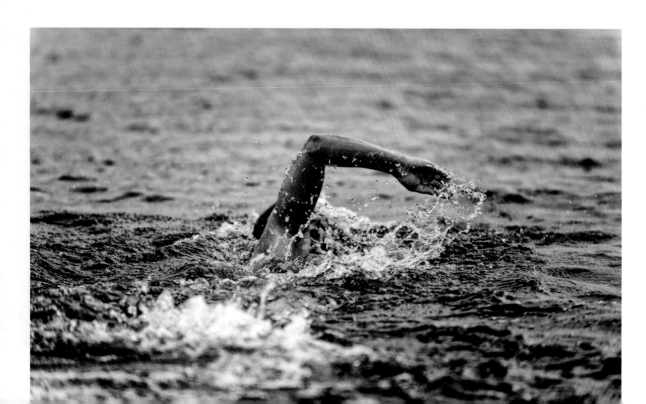

SWIMMING EQUIPMENT

Unless you live in warmer climes, you're going to need a wetsuit sooner or later. Just make sure you try it on for size before you buy. Goggles are essential. Most race organizers insist on a swimming hat, too, and this is normally supplied in the entry pack for the race.

WETSUIT

According to the International Triathlon Union, wetsuits are obligatory for swims up to 1,500m, where the water temperature is below 57°F (14°C), and for swims longer than 1,500m where the water is below 61°F (16°C).

For around $100/£75, you can buy a basic, entry-level wetsuit or you could rent a suit for your first race. Some stores let you buy the suit afterward, discounted by the amount you've spent on the rental. There is, of course, the option of buying a custom-made suit, but this really isn't worth it for a 1,500-m swim.

A word of warning: it's crucial to get the correct fit of wetsuit. If it's too small, you'll feel restricted and won't be able to swim properly; too big and it will cause you to drag in the water. The good news is that many brands now offer up to 15 sizes per style, ensuring that every body, except the most bizarrely shaped, will find a suit that fits perfectly.

Putting on a wetsuit is one of the least graceful acts a triathlete ever has to do. There's honestly no way of doing it with aplomb, but wetsuit lubricant will

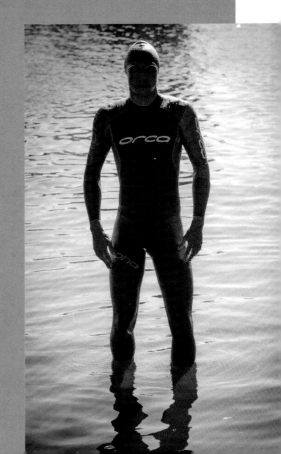

make things easier. Be sure to use specialist lubricant, available from swimwear websites, since petroleum versions can damage your wetsuit. Apply lube to your ankles, lower legs, forearms, wrists, and around your neck. (The latter is to avoid chafing.) Lube will also help you to extricate yourself from the suit after the swim.

Start your wetsuit operation sitting down, so that you don't fall over in front of all the other swimmers. Sit on a towel or mat so you don't damage your suit and remove watches and jewelry for the same reason.

Big-footed swimmers often find it difficult to get their feet into the legs of the wetsuit. One trick is to place plastic bags over your feet before sliding each leg on. Once your legs are in, stand up and gently pull the wetsuit up over your lower body, smoothing out any wrinkles as you go. Don't be too

vigorous: unfortunately some triathlon wetsuits aren't that robust.

Yank the wetsuit too hard, or catch it with a fingernail or toenail, and you risk ripping it. Once your legs are in place, and the suit is pulled right up around your crotch, you can start on your arms. A little bit of wriggling will be required to get your arms fully through and your shoulders in place.

Finally, there's the zipper. All modern triathlon wetsuits feature a zipper at the back. Most zip up from the lower back to the nape of the neck. Some elite wetsuits zip the other way, from the nape of the neck down to the lower back to avoid the tricky situation where another swimmer accidentally pulls your zip lanyard down mid-swim. That would seriously slow your progress. With practice you'll be able to zip up your own suit, but it's best to get a friend or a fellow competitor to do it before the race. Make sure it hangs above the Velcro fastener at the back of your neck so that it doesn't work loose during the swim.

Pro-Tip

Choose the right wetsuit

Mike Trees, ex-pro triathlete and multisport coach

"The more buoyant the wetsuit, the less flexible it is, and vice versa. Unfortunately, a triathlete needs both, but beginners will, on the whole, benefit more from buoyancy than from flexibility. Never buy a suit without wearing it first and, if possible, swim in it before you buy. Some stores with swimming pools or lakes nearby will let you do this. A lot of beginners make the mistake of buying a wetsuit that's too big. This may be comfortable, but when the water gets inside the suit it will slow you down. Ensure that it's a snug fit. The arms below the elbow should be particularly tight, and the neck should be well fitted. Avoid unisex wetsuits because men and women have completely different body shapes."

TRI SUIT

Yes, you can compete with just swimming trunks or a swimsuit beneath your wetsuit, especially if it's a warm-water race, but think about the transitions and the bike and run sections. Do you want to be changing out of your swimsuit in front of hundreds of competitors and spectators? Do you want to be cycling 40km in trunks or a swimsuit?

That's why a tri suit is a really good idea. This is a thin, sleeveless, short-legged (normally Lycra) suit with a chamois crotch that you wear next to your skin beneath your wetsuit. After the swim, you remove your wetsuit and complete the rest of the race in just your tri suit. It means you don't have to run in trunks or a swimsuit (which can seriously chafe!) or waste valuable time changing into new clothing for the bike or run sections. It's quicker, easier, and more professional. You only need a tri suit for race day since you can do all your swimming training in just trunks or a swimsuit, with your wetsuit on top when you need it.

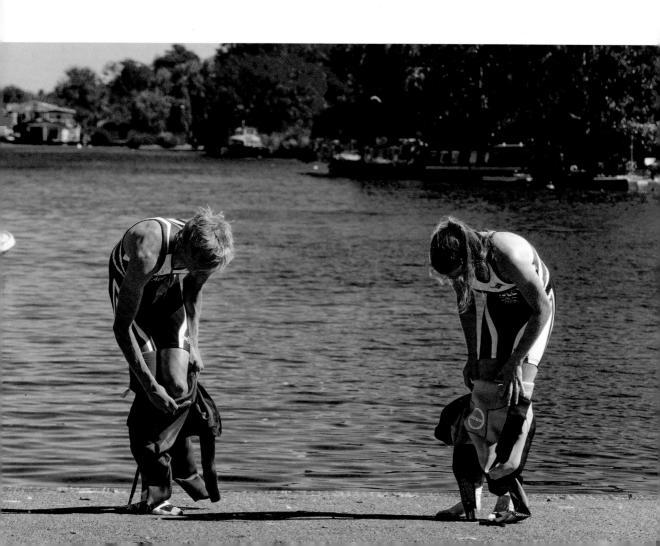

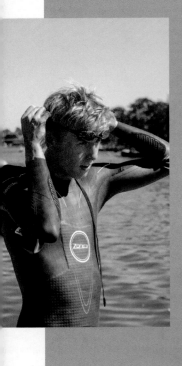

TIP: Don't spit in your goggles right after eating food, otherwise your last mouthful will be swimming around in front of your eyes!

GOGGLES

It's worth spending a bit of money on quality goggles that fit you properly. You'll wish you had when you're trying to tread water in "the washing machine" (see page 118), furiously adjusting your goggles while the other swimmers are thrashing around you.

Always try before you buy and remember that a good fit is determined by the seal, not the strap. When you press the goggles to your eyes (without putting on the strap), the seal should hold them in place for a few seconds. They should adhere comfortably to the orbit around your eyes—not too loose or they'll let in water, and not too tight or they'll put pressure on your face. Split straps hold goggles in place better; don't over-tighten the straps. Opt for a brand with anti-fogging treatment and UV protection. If you're swimming only in open water, you could try a swimming mask, which is bigger than goggles but not as big as a snorkeling mask.

When it comes to lens color, consider where and when you'll be swimming. Clear lenses are great for indoor swimming; amber lenses enhance vision in low light; mirrored lenses reduce glare from the sun and the water, and so are perfect for outdoor swimming in summer. If you're short-sighted, you may need to splash out on prescription lenses for your goggles.

Always keep your goggles in a bag or box so they don't get scratched.

Even the most expensive goggles will start to fog up over time. There are many fluids you can rub on the inside of the lenses to prevent this, with mixed results: saliva, anti-fogging spray, baby shampoo, shaving cream, toothpaste, dishwashing liquid. Find out which one works best for you.

SWIM HAT

A swim hat will keep your head warm, keep your hair out of your eyes, streamline your head, and ensure you can be spotted in the water. Triathlons with open-water swimming often supply race hats to all competitors. Get used to wearing one during your training swims.

SWIM TRAINING AIDS

At the pool you might see experienced swimmers employing all sorts of training aids: leg bands, pull buoys, fins, paddles, floats. Don't worry yourself too much about these. Concentrate on finessing your front crawl and your swimming drills. To use swim training aids properly, you'll likely need the advice of a qualified coach or a friend who has good swimming expertise.

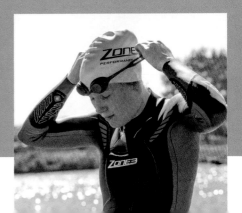

TRIATHLON LEGENDS
Alistair Brownlee (Great Britain)

BORN: April 23, 1988, Dewsbury, UK

OLYMPIC GAMES GOLD MEDAL: London 2012, Rio 2016

ITU WORLD CHAMPION: 2009, 2011

Jonathan Brownlee (Great Britain)

BORN: April 30, 1990, Dewsbury, UK

OLYMPIC GAMES SILVER MEDAL: Rio 2016

OLYMPIC GAMES BRONZE MEDAL: London 2012

ITU WORLD CHAMPION: 2012

These outstanding triathletes are the first British brothers ever to finish first and second in an Olympic event. Between them the Brownlee brothers have four Olympic medals, four Commonwealth Games medals, and over a dozen World Championship medals.

Hailing from West Yorkshire, UK, the brothers currently live just down the road from each other in a village in the northern suburbs of Leeds, making joint training sessions easy to organize.

However much they end up achieving in their careers, they will surely be remembered forever for that moment in 2016 when, during a World Series race in Mexico, Alistair sacrificed first place to help his heat-exhausted brother, on the verge of collapse, across the finish line.

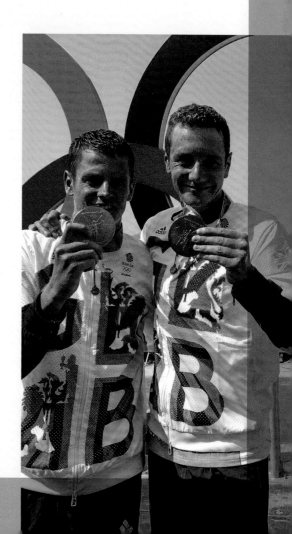

SWIMMING TECHNIQUES

Start off working on your swimming technique in a swimming pool. Once you've built up a bit of confidence, you can make the move to open water. If you're really apprehensive about your technique, you might want to pay for a few swimming lessons.

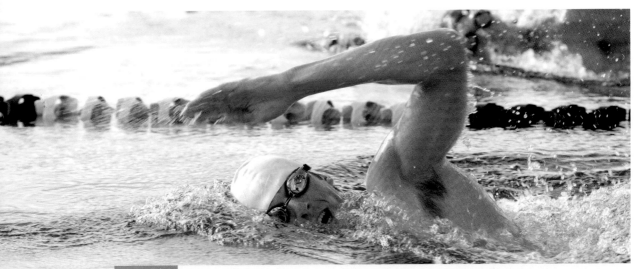

Pro-Tip

Breathing tips

<u>Paul Newsome, head coach at swimming coaching company Swim Smooth</u>

"Work on your bilateral breathing (i.e. breathing on both sides as you swim). It will improve the symmetry of your swimming. Simply say the words 'bubble, bubble, breathe, bubble, bubble, breathe...' over and over again as you exhale in the water and alternate breathing on both sides. This mantra will help you control some of the anxiety you're likely to experience when you swim your first strokes in open water.

"When you're breathing on the front crawl, do your best Popeye impression: one eye stays in the water, and one eye emerges, while your mouth is angled like you're chewing spinach. This helps keep your head low and your body profile effective in the water."

FRONT CRAWL

Yes, in theory, you can swim your first triathlon using breaststroke or even doggy paddle. But have some pride, won't you, and adopt the front crawl. You don't have to perform it like some sort of Michael Phelps. It can be slow. It can be ugly. But do yourself a favor and make it your mission to complete your first triathlon swim with 100 percent front crawl. Here are some basic tips:

≡ Keep your body flat and parallel with the water surface as you swim. Drop your legs too much and you create unnecessary drag.

≡ Roll your torso slightly from side to side with each stroke. Your stomach and core muscles should be tight to support your lower back.

≡ Position your head so your face is looking down toward the bottom of the pool. Raise your eyes so you can see where you're heading.

≡ Keep your legs close together. Move your whole leg from the hip downward when you kick, but keep the kick movements small and beneath the surface of the water. Kick your legs alternately and with your legs as straight as possible. Remember that kicking is to maintain stability in the water, not for propulsion.

≡ For the arm movements, start by pointing one elbow to the sky. Then push your hand into the water about 18in (45cm) in front of you, in line with your shoulder. Fully extend the arm before pulling it down and back in an S-shape all the way to your hips, catching as much water as possible as you do so. Finish the arm movement by bringing your arm close to your body so you are as streamlined as possible.

≡ When you breathe, don't lift your entire head out of the water because your legs will sink and you'll create drag. One side of your face should remain submerged as you breathe. How often you breathe and whether you breathe on one side or both is entirely up to you. But if you're swimming in open water, you should train yourself to breathe on both sides. This helps you deal with waves, spot landmarks, and monitor rival swimmers.

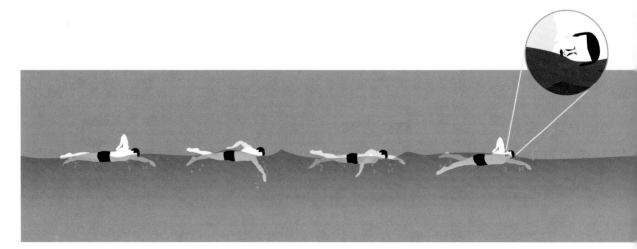

Here are some great remedies to reduce your drag:

≡ Slightly rotate the long axis of your spine with each stroke as you swim. Being too flat makes it hard for your arms to recover over the top of the water, but equally rotating too much causes you to lose balance and your legs to splay apart.

≡ For many newer swimmers, looking down in the water is a way to keep your legs higher and reduce drag. But for some swimmers in wetsuits, looking too far down can be problematic and unbalancing.

≡ Don't kick your legs too hard. Even the great Ian Thorpe only generated 11 percent of his entire propulsion from his leg kick. For triathletes, extended legs, loose floppy ankles, and toes that brush against each other with each kick are ideal for reducing drag and not wasting too much energy.

≡ Aim to enter the water finger-tips first and then push a straight line back toward your hips as though you are pulling yourself along an imaginary rope.

Touch turn

The easiest way to turn at the end of each lane is a method called the touch turn. Beginners do a basic version of this naturally without even thinking about it, but there are ways to streamline it

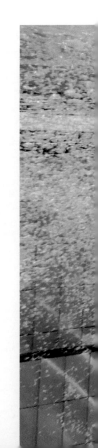

Pro-Tip

Reduce drag in the water

<u>Paul Newsome, head coach at Swim Smooth</u>

Many swimmers feel their legs drag behind them when they swim. Efficient swimming is all about trying to reduce drag and increase propulsion to ensure you're both smooth and speedy at the same time. Drag might occur for the following reasons:

1. You're holding onto your breath, making you more buoyant at the front.

2. You're moving your arms across the front of your head, causing your body to snake around in the water and your legs to scissor apart.

3. You're pushing down on the water with your arms to lift you high up in order to breathe.

4. You're kicking excessively from the knee and with stiff ankles.

5. You're looking too far forward when your head is down in the water and not breathing.

and win a few milliseconds on each turn. (Over the course of a pool race that can add up to a few seconds' advantage.)

After your final stroke of each length, glide to the end of the lane with one arm extended. Swing your legs beneath your torso and place the balls of both feet against the wall, a couple of feet below the surface, one above the other. Once you've turned your body, lift your head out of the water and take a deep breath. Now drop down so your head and body are fully submerged, your arms are fully extended, and you're pointing back up the lane you've just swum down. Simultaneously, use both legs to push away from the wall. Your body will be parallel with the pool floor, but slightly

on its side. Your arms and hands should remain fully extended in the diving position, with your head tucked between your arms.

It's now that patience is crucial. As you glide away from the wall, turning from your side onto your front, remain submerged for as long as you continue gliding. Don't start kicking yet. Depending on how hard your push-off was, you could continue gliding underwater for as much as 5m (15ft). Toward the end of the glide, gradually rise to the surface before breathing and starting your first stroke. Continue swimming normally.

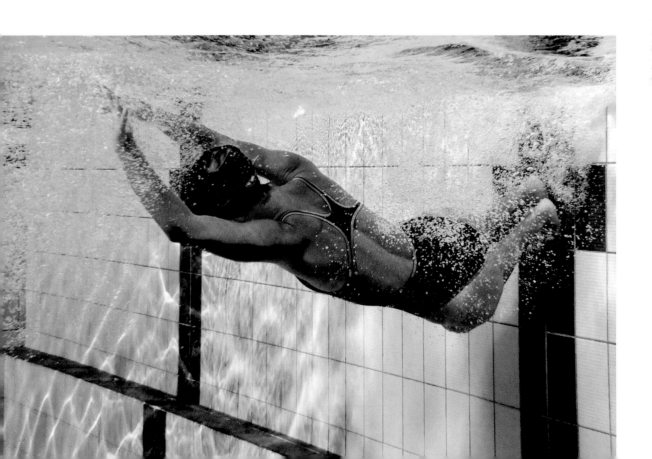

Tumble turn

Even some seasoned triathletes don't bother to learn the tumble turn. After all, if all their competitive swimming is done in open water, why bother? But it's got to be said: the tumble turn is really cool. It will impress other pool users and make you feel like you're making real progress in your swim training. It will also make your training sessions much smoother. If you've got the time to practice it, then why not adopt it as part of your normal swimming technique? Don't fear the tumble turn. Here's how to do it:

≡ A couple of feet before you reach the end of the pool, execute a forward somersault, tucking your chin into your chest and your legs up to your backside. Don't twist your body yet. Make sure you exhale throughout the entire somersault to stop water going up your nose.

≡ Place your feet on the wall, with your legs still tucked up to your backside. Push off hard from the wall, extending your arms straight and your palms facing downward.

≡ Twist your body so that you rotate from a face-up position to a face-down position.

≡ Glide in a streamlined position for as long as you can. Dolphin kicks will keep you gliding farther.

≡ Rise to the surface and start your first stroke as your head breaks the surface.

Pro-Tip

The pros and cons of tumble turns

Paul Newsome, head coach at Swim Smooth

Pros:

1. Ultimately, it's the fastest way to turn because of the mechanics of the turn and the greater in-out spring effect off the wall.

2. A fast turn means you can stay with swimmers who would otherwise be slightly faster than yourself—useful in a squad training situation. Done well, a tumble is perhaps as much as 0.3–0.5 seconds faster than a good touch turn.

3. It's easier to execute on a high-walled pool without a gutter.

4. You look like a real swimmer.

Cons:

1. Tumbling can be challenging to learn. It's disorientating at first. Water can easily go up your nose. You can't take a breath during the turn, which makes things harder aerobically, especially when swimming hard over distance.

2. It requires a supple back.

SWIMMING DRILLS

Swimming endless lengths up and down the pool will eventually bore you senseless—even professional swimmers get bored by lengths. To break up the monotony of all that training, you need a few swimming drills.

KICK-ON-THE-SIDE DRILL

Learning to kick on your side is a staple component of a good front-crawl stroke. Swim a length on one side with your lower arm outstretched, your upper arm by your side, and your eyes looking to the bottom of the pool. Keep your body on its side and maintain a good posture in the water, with your shoulders back and your chest forward. Your lead palm should be facing straight down to the bottom of the pool, holding you firm as you kick. When you breathe, tilt your head to the side. Avoid the temptation to push down with your lead arm in order to lift your head out of the water. On alternate lengths, switch to the other side of your body.

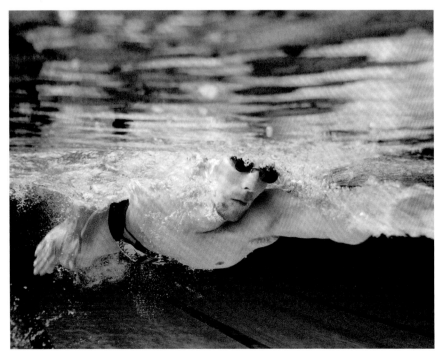

6/1/6 DRILL

Once you've mastered kick-on-the-side drills, it's time to make things a bit more dynamic. Start exactly as you did with the kick-on-the-side drill. Hold that position for six kicks, and then make a front-crawl stroke so that your body rotates over onto its other side. Take a breath as your head rolls round. Repeat the same sequence on the other side. You will end up putting together a sequence of six kicks, one stroke, six kicks—hence the name 6/1/6.

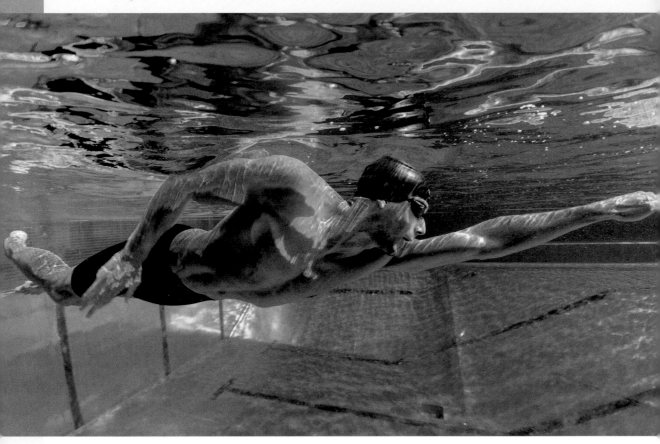

CATCH-UP STROKE

Keep your left arm fully outstretched until your right arm has come forward and joined it in the outstretched position. Now leave your right arm fully outstretched until your left arm has stroked forward to join it. Swimming like this encourages you to reach out fully during your stroke, and makes your swimming style smoother and more efficient, saving you energy.

DRAFTING DRILLS

Get a group of three or more swimmers together. While you swim lengths of the pool, take turns leading the group and drafting at the back of the group. Switch positions every couple of lengths. (See page 44 for drafting tips.)

SIGHTING DRILLS

Swim your normal front crawl, but with your head up and eyes permanently raised out of the water as if you were sighting. (See page 44 for sighting tips.) This will train you for sighting during an open-water swim. Do this drill only for short distances.

OPEN-WATER SWIMMING

GETTING STARTED

It's possible this is your first experience of swimming in a tri suit and/or a wetsuit. If so, get acclimatized. First walk into the lake up to your chest. Splash your head and face with water. Undo your wetsuit collar and splash a bit of water inside. Feel the water warm up as it enters the suit and gets close to your skin.

Now practice treading water. Get used to the unusual sensation of being in a deep lake. Lie flat on the surface of the water, both face down and face up. Feel the water around you. Allow lake weed to touch you in the face. You're going to be swimming through a lot of weed during your open-water training.

Now practice a few strokes. It will feel very strange since, in a triathlon-specific wetsuit (don't use anything designed for other water sports—it just won't cut the mustard), you're more buoyant but slightly constricted in your movements. The constriction around the shoulders, in particular, means you'll need to rotate your upper body slightly more than when you're in just your trunks or swimsuit. But the extra buoyancy is a bonus since it brings you closer to the surface, reducing drag as you swim through the water. Even the best professional swimmers struggle to swim in a perfectly straight line. Most of us have one side of the body stronger than the other. Over the course of several hundred meters, this can cause you to veer off course if you're not careful, adding unnecessarily to your overall distance.

SAFETY FIRST: A word of warning: only swim in a lake that is geared up for open-water swimming. You will normally have to pay a small fee; and supervisors will be present during opening hours, which is reassuring if you are a weak swimmer. You can be sure the water will be clean, too. On your first few lake swims, for your own confidence, bring along a more experienced friend.

Here are some tips on how to swim fast and straight in open water:

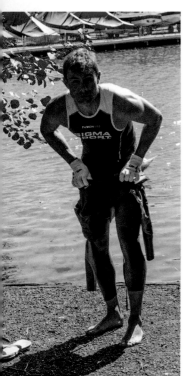

Put your wetsuit on properly

Pull the wetsuit high up into your crotch, and fully up your legs and arms so it's not so restrictive around the shoulders. This will free up your shoulders, allowing you to make freer strokes.

Swim symmetrically

Concentrate on applying equal power with both arms, and catching the same amount of water on both sides. Symmetry will keep you in a straight line.

Breathe efficiently

Despite the unfamiliar environment, learn to inhale and exhale fully while you're swimming. This will help you overcome any anxiety on the race day. If you find you're veering markedly off to one side, it might be because you breathe only to one side. Rectify this by learning to breathe on both sides (bilateral breathing). Whether you do this every three or five strokes is up to you. Whatever feels most natural. Bilateral breathing isn't for everyone, though. If you really can't make it work, then stick with breathing on one side.

Sight effectively

If you want to swim straight, you need to master the fine skill of sighting. Proper sighting involves raising your head to look where you're going—using a buoy or a prominent landmark on dry land as your guide—but without slowing your progress too much. Time your sighting so that you do it just before you're due to breathe. Press down on the water surface with your leading arm, and lift just your eyes out of the water (not your whole head) for a split second to see where you're going. As you lower your head, turn your head sideways into its normal breathing position and carry on swimming. This should ensure you retain your rhythm.

Save time by drafting

Drafting is when you swim just a few inches directly behind a swimmer, or slightly behind and to the side of them. (The latter is called hip drafting.) Essentially you're swimming in the slipstream created by the swimmer in front. It means you can swim as fast as normal, but without expending as much energy. Experts reckon drafting can save between 18–25 percent of the energy you'd normally use. That's energy you can use later on, so make the most of it.

Triathlon beginners are understandably nervous about drafting, for fear of being kicked in the face. It's a technique you should practice with your friends first so you know how to gauge the correct distance between you and the person you're drafting: close but not too close. If you choose to draft to the side of another swimmer, it's best to turn your head toward them when you breathe. This allows you to keep an eye on their position, and stops you colliding.

TRIATHLON LEGENDS
Mark Allen (USA)

BORN:	January 12, 1958, Glendale, California, USA
IRONMAN WORLD CHAMPION:	1989–1993, 1995
ITU WORLD CHAMPION:	1989

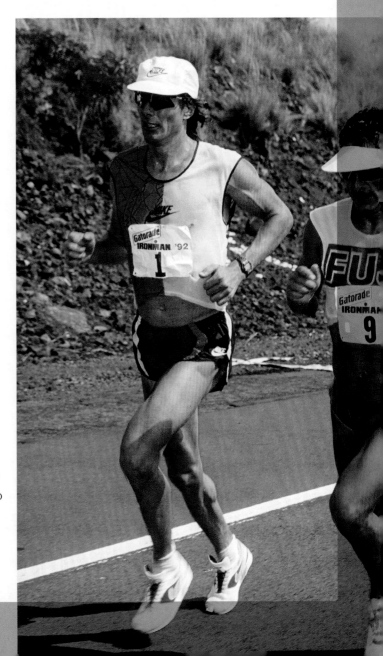

Back in 1982, Mark Allen was watching highlights of the Ironman Hawaii on television. That was the year Julie Moss collapsed 400 meters from the end of the race and famously crawled her way across the finish line. Allen was so moved by the incident (to tears, in fact) that he decided to enter the very next Ironman event the same year.

It was the start of a stellar career that eventually saw him winning a staggering six Ironman championships, as well as triathlon's inaugural World Championships in 1989. Much of his competition was defined by his rivalry with fellow American triathlete Dave Scott.

And that television footage of Julie Moss's crawl across the finish line obviously moved him in more ways than one since he ended up being married to her from 1989 to 2002!

CHAPTER 3

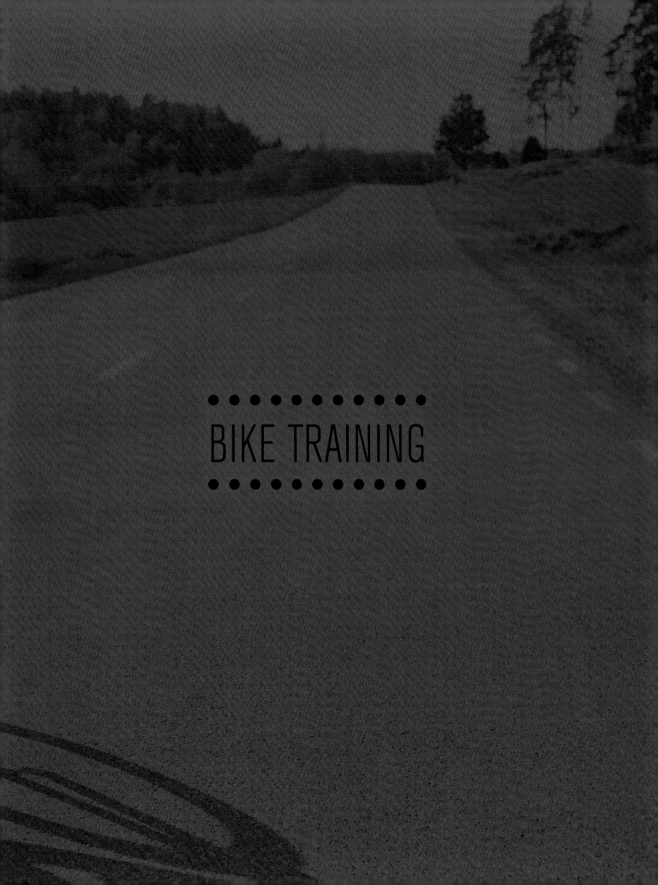

BIKE TRAINING

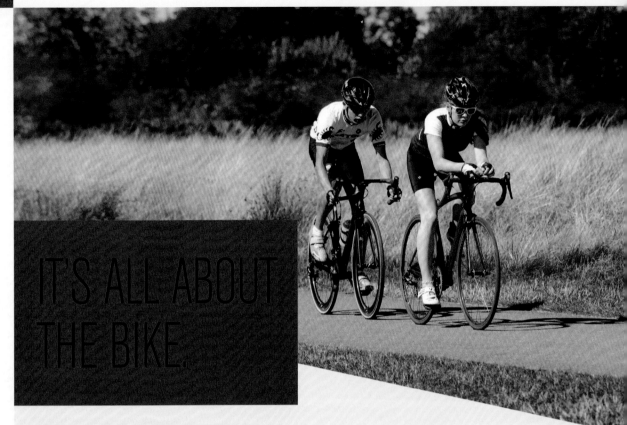

IT'S ALL ABOUT THE BIKE.

This is the one triathlon discipline where equipment (and the maintenance of it) can make a serious difference to your overall time. For that reason, you need to know your way round your bike. But don't, whatever you do, stress too much about the brand, model, or quality of bike you're racing on, especially if you're only doing a Sprint race.

At an entry-level Sprint triathlon you'll see all sorts of dilapidated bikes on show: cheap mountain bikes with off-road tires still on them; old-school racing bikes from the 1980s; hybrids that look barely suitable for a trip to the local store, let alone a race. Remember, the Sprint-distance bike section is only 20km. If your budget is tight and you're not even sure yet whether triathlon is really the sport for you, you can complete 20km on a fairly low-quality machine, as long as it's properly maintained (see pages 58–60). Yes, you'll be slower than someone on a three-grand carbon-frame road bike, but over such a short distance, you won't be that much slower.

HYBRID/STREET BIKE

These bikes aren't designed for competition, but rather for commuting or general street riding. Yes, you can happily complete your first triathlon on a hybrid—and there will be other beginners on these bikes—but you won't post a particularly fast time. And, crucially, you won't look like you're committed to the sport.

MOUNTAIN BIKE

These are designed for cycling off-road, hence the stronger, less aerodynamic frames. If you use one in your first race, make sure you replace the off-road tires with slick tires—the narrowest slicks that your wheel rims can accommodate. This will save you more than a few seconds over the entire bike section. As with hybrid bikes, you won't look like you're a committed triathlete.

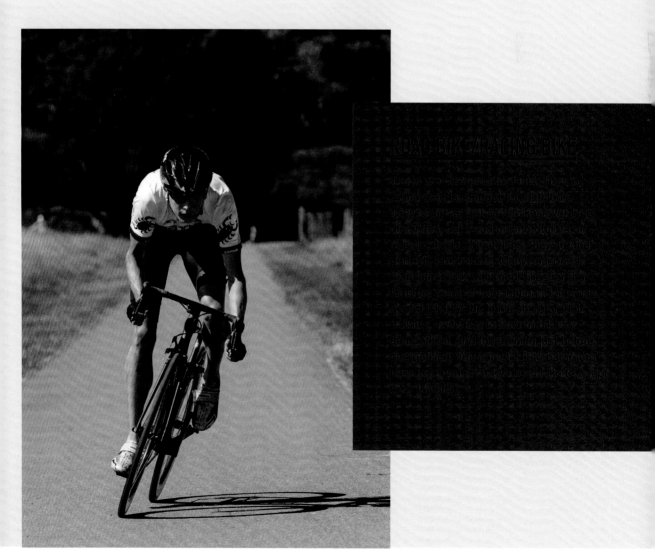

ROAD BIKE / RACING BIKE

These are designed for racing, and they are faster and lighter over long distances than the mountain or hybrid. If you complete your first triathlon on a road bike, you will look committed. You will pull out of transition quicker, too. Buy or borrow a road bike for competition, and train hard just before competition. You'll get the best over the race track—which equals a decent race time.

TRI BIKE

Specifically designed for triathlon competition, these are the best bikes you can buy for the price of the top-end models, you can spend the same as you would on a decent car. Tri bikes are for serious triathletes. They feature tri bars/aero bars, aerodynamic wheels, sometimes with tri spokes, knife-thin saddles, extra-thin profile frames, and a frame geometry designed for the ultimate aerodynamic riding position. Be warned, if you turn up for your first Sprint triathlon with a 10-grand tri bike, you will be universally mocked. There's a common expression in triathlon—"all the gear and no idea." Don't buy a tri bike unless you plan to dedicate much of your free time to triathlon. It's simply not worth it.

Pro-Tip

Choice of bike

Jonathan Brownlee, triathlon champion

"Train and do your first race (on your existing bike) before you buy an expensive bike. See if you enjoy the sport. You can always adapt your existing bike—even if it's a mountain bike with slicks on it. If you really enjoy it, then you can buy a faster bike later on."

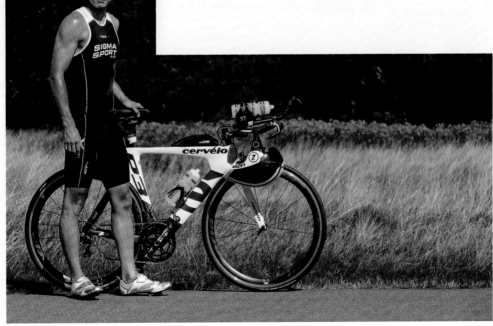

ANATOMY OF A BIKE

Let's assume you've managed to beg, borrow, or steal a road bike for your first triathlon. (Actually, don't steal it; that would be really bad Karma.) Get to know your bike inside out, well in advance of the race.

KNOWING THE BASICS

Before you start training on your bike, make sure the saddle, seat post, and handlebars are set up correctly for your height. Learn your way round the gears and the brakes. Ensure your tires are pumped to the correct pressure, and keep checking them. Teach yourself how to lubricate your chainset and change an inner tube quickly and efficiently. If you suffer a puncture during a Sprint or Olympic triathlon, you'll slow your overall time substantially, but you should still be able to replace your inner tube and finish the race.

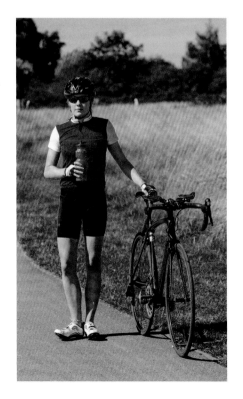

WHAT SIZE FRAME?

Be sure to get the correct size of frame if you're buying a new bike. Traditionally, road bikes are measured in centimeters (since Europe is the spiritual home of the road bike), while mountain bikes are measure in inches (since USA is the spiritual home of the mountain bike). But, to make things confusing, different manufacturers from different parts of the world measure their bikes in different ways.

One general guideline is this: stand astride the bike, one leg either side of the top tube. There should be 2in (5cm) between your crotch and the top of the top tube. You also need to take into account your reach so that you're not too stretched out nor too hunched up when your arms are on the handlebars.

Average women have longer legs and shorter torsos than average men of the same height. This explains why some bike models are manufactured as female-specific with shorter top tubes. To accommodate the female body, they may also have narrower handlebars and differently shaped saddles.

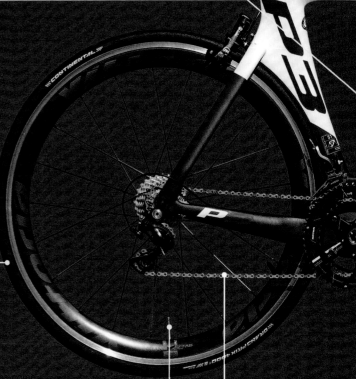

Saddle

You're going to spend a lot of time on your ride during training. If you don't adjust it for comfort and efficiency, you're going to suffer. Once you've found it, adjust First, set the saddle at the correct height. If you're too low, you waste energy; too high and you can't pedal smoothly. When your leg is fully extended, make sure your knee is slightly bent.

Now for the saddle position, using a hex key (Allen key), you can change the position – forwards or back. Try to do so to make it more comfortable. It all depends on your personal anatomy, and only you can be the judge of that.

Water bottles

Make sure you have at least one water bottle cage on your bike frame. For Sprint triathlons you'll need only one cage. For Olympic distance you might need two.

Tires

Keep your tires at the correct pressure and you'll increase your speed round the course. But how much pressure depends on your weight, the width of your tires, and the road surface. Ideally, an 190lb (86kg) rider should inflate tires to around 90lb per square inch (6 bars). Nearly every tire has the recommended range of pressure printed on its side wall. By inflating it below or above this range, you risk losing control of the bike on corners or degrading the tire more quickly than usual. As you increase the tire pressure, you reduce friction with the road surface, but you also reduce the traction.

Valves

There are three main types of valves. Most road bikes and triathlons come with Presta valves (the thinner type that have a screw-top beneath the cap). Mountain bikes come with either Presta or Schrader valves. The latter are larger, the same as motor car tire valves. The third type is called a Dunlop valve. Learn how your valves work on your bike, so you can inflate your tires quickly before and during your race.

Chain

Keep your chain lubricated, clean, and in good condition to prolong the life of the chain.

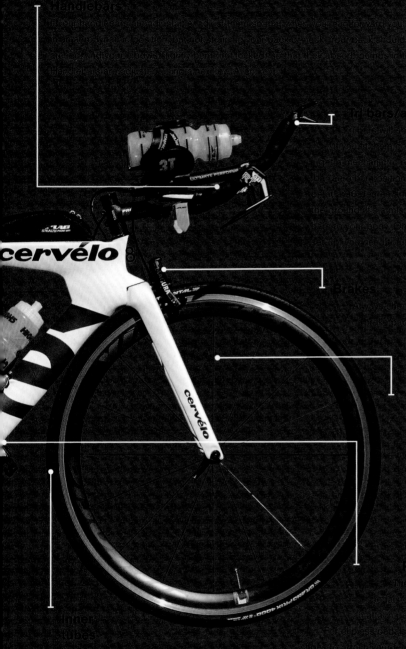

Handlebars

The standard bars are adjustable so that you can set up your bike how you see fit. In a good pursuit position when you're on your bike the back should be straight and your elbows slightly bent so that it acts as a shock absorber in the road. Handlebars are relatively long, providing a lot of leverage.

Tri bars/aero bars

These will shave a valuable few seconds off your bike ride, but only if you use them correctly. They aren't always easy to use ideally, so get used to them if you plan to use them with your bike. When in the aero position, your upper arms should be vertical and your forearms horizontal, your lower arms parallel. The idea is to transfer all your body to the bars, rather than the back of your neck. Once you've found you feel comfortable in bars, make sure you get used to using them on your training rides.

Brakes

Always check your brakes are functioning properly and that the wheels stop when you apply the brake levers when pressed.

Spokes

Spokes can become loose, this can cause your wheel to buckle. You will need to straighten up your wheel, tighten up any loose spokes using a spoke key. This can be rather complicated and it is easy to inadvertently tighten the spokes you need to loosen, and vice versa, so watch instructional videos online first.

Pedal

There are two types of pedal: flat and clipless. Flat pedals can be used with normal running shoes. You would then strap your shoes to flat pedals for extra pedal power. For clipless pedals you need cleats on the bottom of your cycling shoes that attach yourself securely to the pedals. There are two types of clipless pedals, some are so that you can walk in since the cleats are recessed into your shoes and others where the cleats aren't recessed. Over the course of a race, clipless pedals will save you a substantial amount of time as they allow you to pedal more efficiently, and to drive the pedals with an upward motion as well as down. You may need to put in a bit of practice to get used to them, however. Expect to wobble a little the first few times you use them. Once you've got used to them, though, they will become natural to you and you'll never turn back.

Inner tubes

If you get a puncture during a race it's vital that you can change the inner tube quickly. Inner tubes are relatively quick and easy to replace, once you know how. Practice changing your inner tube at home so that you won't be wasting precious time on the course.

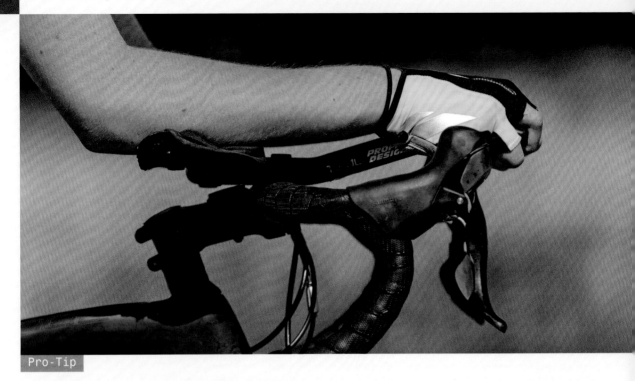

Pro-Tip

Get the right tri bars/aero bars

Steve Lumley, Malaysia-based triathlon coach

"Your upper arm should be at a 90-degree angle to the ground, with your elbows directly under your shoulders. Your forearms should then be parallel to the ground. This position will ensure you can ride comfortably without having to grip onto the bars with your hands.

"If you can't get an effective and comfortable position without compromising your saddle and pedaling position, then you may well have the wrong bars, or the wrong bike, or both. The best riding position is if your back is close to being parallel with the ground. Just a few degrees raised from this, in fact. But don't adopt this position at the expense of your comfort. If you can't ride like that for at least an hour, or it compromises pedaling power, then it's not going to be good in a race situation.

"Get used to being in that position for extended periods of time. As much as possible, your training in the eight weeks prior to the race should emulate what you will actually be doing in the race."

TRIATHLON LEGENDS
Jan Frodeno (Germany)

BORN:	August 18, 1981, Cologne, Germany
OLYMPIC GAMES GOLD MEDAL:	Beijing 2008
IRONMAN WORLD CHAMPION:	2015, 2016

It was while living in South Africa, as a teenager, that German-born Frodeno first got seriously involved in sport, but only as a swimmer, not a triathlete. Then in 2000, he started honing his skills in all three triathlon disciplines, returning to his native Germany where he trained as part of the national triathlon team. By 2015, he had made history by becoming the first triathlete, male or female, to win both a gold medal in the Olympic triathlon and the Ironman World Championship title.

He is married to Emma Snowsill who, like him, won triathlon gold at the Beijing Olympics.

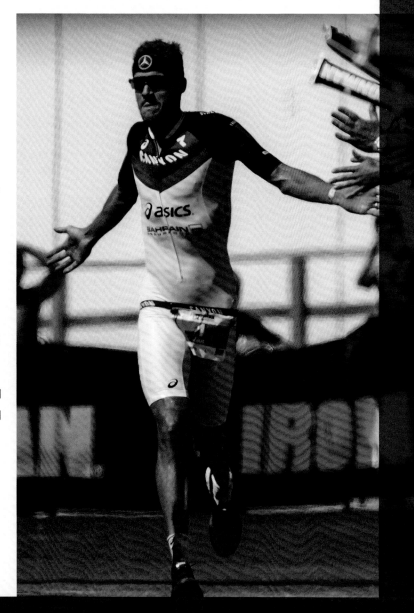

OTHER BIKE EQUIPMENT

Cyclists often go overboard on all the bike accessories they buy. And at every triathlon race you'll spot plenty of competitors who look like they've got all the gear but no idea. Saying that, there are certain accessories that you can't do without—a helmet being the most essential of all.

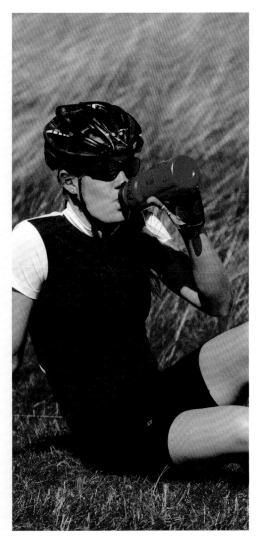

CYCLE CLOTHING

During the race you'll be cycling in either your trunks or swimsuit with a T-shirt on top, or in your tri suit (see page 33). But for all those miles of training on the bike you'll need Lycra cycle shorts (with a chamois insert), a cycling jersey (with rear pockets), and a windproof cycling jacket (also with rear pockets). All cycling clothing now comes in materials that wick away the sweat.

CYCLING EYEWEAR

Cycle down a dusty road in the summer and you'll quickly realize that eyewear is vital to protect your eyes. Unless you particularly like having grit and insects swimming around your eyeballs, that is. Some cycling glasses feature interchangeable lenses with cloudy day, sunny day, and light-enhancing lens options. Bear in mind that your cycling glasses are going to get spattered with rain, mud, gravel, bugs, and exhaust fumes. You'll drop them every now and then. At the end of your training rides you'll throw them into your kitbag. Sooner or later you'll step on them. Fall for the advertising and you'll end up spending a week's wages on all-singing, all-dancing cycling glasses. There's no reason why you can't get away with cheap eyewear on the bike, as long as they carry a CE or FCC mark. (Different territories have different safety standards.)

CYCLING GLOVES

Fall off your bike and it's often your palms that hit the deck first. Gloves both protect your palms and keep your hands warm. You'll need a fingerless pair for summer training and a warmer, full-fingered pair for winter.

NUMBER BELT

For most triathlon races you'll have to wear an elastic race belt to which you attach your race number. Never wear a race number during training, though. That's very sad.

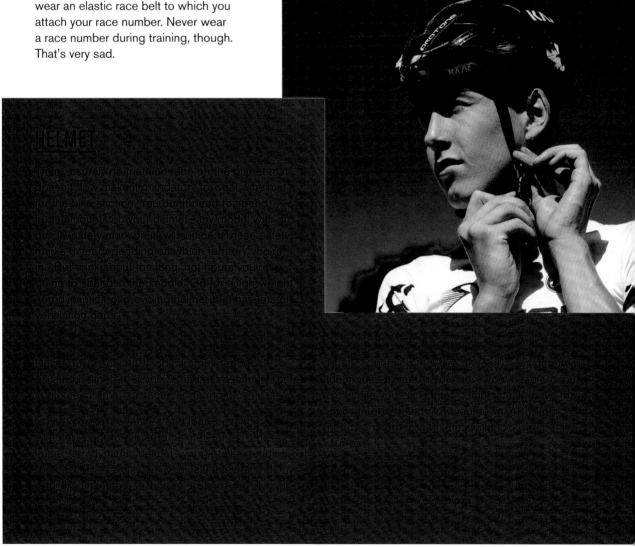

HELMET

There's surely no triathlon race on the planet that doesn't now make it mandatory to wear a helmet for the bike section. You don't need to spend huge amounts on your helmet—any model with an official safety mark on it will suffice. These safety marks differ depending on which territory you're in. But think about the long, hot hours you're going to spend in the saddle. Go for a lightweight, aerodynamic road cycling helmet that has lots of ventilation gaps.

BASIC BIKE REPAIRS

With all the bike training you'll be doing, there is sure to come a time when you'll need to do some basic roadside repairs. Sod's Law says this will be when you're the farthest distance from home or a bike repair store as possible. And the sun's going down and it's started raining.

TOOLS YOU NEED

All the essential tools you'll need out on your bike ride will fit easily into a small bag. You can mount the pump onto your frame.

Puncture repair kit
A traditional puncture repair kit includes tire levers, glue, patches, sandpaper, and chalk. But it's fiddly. Use glueless patches instead as these are much easier to work with. You'll still need tire levers to get the tire on and off.

Multi-tool
This will include basic spanners, hex keys (Allen keys), and a screwdriver. Some also include a chain tool (see below).

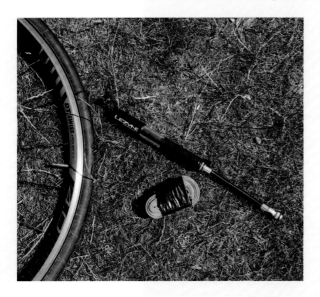

Spare inner tube
Some punctures are irreparable. The hole might be too big, for example, or the valve might split from the tube. In these cases, you'll need a new inner tube.

Pump
Make sure you have the correct adaptor for your valves. There are two types: Schrader is the fatter one, also used on cars. Presta is the thinner one. Most road bikes come with Presta valves. Mountain bikes come with either Presta or Schrader.

Chain tool
Without this it's impossible to fix a broken chain.

HOW TO CLEAN AND LUBRICATE YOUR CHAIN

As you ride, your chain picks up lots of mud and dirt from the roads and trails. It will need regular cleaning and lubricating.

1. Turn your bike upside down so that it is balancing on its handlebars and saddle.

2. Scrape any mud or dirt from the cogs and the derailleurs.

3. Grasp the chain with a rag and press tight.

4. Turn the pedals (backward is easier) with one hand so that the chain revolves and grime comes off the chain onto the rag.

5. Still turning the pedals with one hand, spray or drizzle your lubricant onto the chain as it goes through the rear derailleur, making sure you coat the entire chain. Not too much and not too little. Ensure you don't inadvertently get lubricant on the brakes.

6. Now run through the gears to disperse the lubricant evenly. Finally, run the chain through a rag once again to wipe off any excess.

HOW TO REPLACE A CHAIN THAT'S SLIPPED OFF

Every once in a while, the chain will slip off the cogs. It's simple to replace it.

1. Lift up the chain and hook it onto the smallest sprocket at the front of the chainset.

2. Holding the rear wheel off the ground, use your hand to pedal the chain backward. Then, again using your hand, pedal forward until the chain slips into the correct gear position.

3. Sometimes the chain gets jammed between the smallest rear cog and rear triangle. If this happens, loosen the quick-release lever on the wheel. Lift up the chain and place it back on the cogs. Re-tighten the quick-release lever before using your hand to pedal the chain back into its correct gear position.

HOW TO FIX A PUNCTURE

It's essential to know how to repair a puncture. Here's a step-by-step guide:

1. Remove the wheel from the forks (if it's the front wheel that's punctured) or from the drop-outs (if it's the rear wheel). If it's not a quick-release wheel, you'll need a spanner for this.

2. Use tire levers to get the tire off the wheel. Insert the first tire lever between the tire and wheel rim. Gently bend it back, pry the tire beading from the rim, and hook the other end of the tire lever to one of your spokes. Insert the second lever 2in (5cm) farther round the tire. Remove the first lever and place it another 2in (5cm) farther round the tire. Eventually, one side of the tire will come away from the wheel. (This is tougher with new tires since they have a tighter fit.)

3. Starting with the valve, remove the inner tube from the wheel. Using your fingers, check the tire—both inside and outside—for thorns or pieces of glass.

4. Inflate the tube with your pump. Pass the tube over your lips so that you can feel even the smallest leak of air. When you locate the puncture hole, keep your finger on it so you don't forget where it is. Often you can align the tube with the tire so as to find the cause of the puncture.

5. Roughen the puncture hole with the sandpaper in your repair kit. Apply glue to the area around the hole and leave to dry for at least a minute. Stick on the patch too early and it won't seal. (Glueless patches are much easier to apply.)

6. Press the patch firmly over the hole and leave to dry.

7. Slightly inflate the tube and place it back into the tire. Put the valve back into the wheel's rim hole. Use your fingers to work one edge of the tire back into the wheel rim, and then as much of the second edge as you can. Eventually the tire will be so tight that you'll need levers to insert the final section. Be extra careful not to pinch the tube as you do this or you may cause another puncture.

8. Fully inflate the tire and re-attach the wheel to the forks or drop-outs.

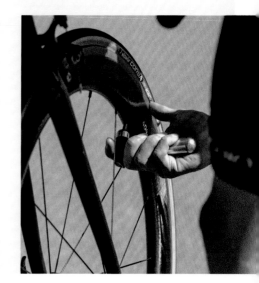

TRIATHLON LEGENDS
Natascha Badmann (Switzerland)

BORN: December 6, 1966, Basel, Switzerland

IRONMAN WORLD CHAMPION: 1998, 2000–2002, 2004, 2005

When Switzerland's Natascha Badmann won the Ironman World Championships in 1998, she was the first European woman to do so. There had been podium places for a Briton, a Dutchwoman, and a French woman before her, but never in first place. It was the start of a purple patch that saw her win the title a total of six times.

What makes this Swiss athlete's achievements all the more impressive is that, during her 20s, as she admits, she was an "overweight, smoking secretary" with a daughter to take care of. Not the typical base on which to build a top-level triathlon career. In fact, with the help of a work colleague called Toni Hasler, Badmann turned her life around. Spotting her raw potential, Hasler became her coach, nutritionist, and eventually her husband.

Badmann now works in Switzerland as a social worker.

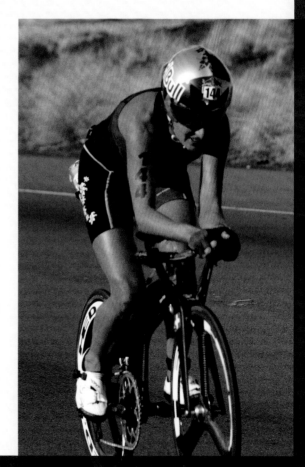

BIKE HANDLING SKILLS

Road cyclists and mountain bikers like to joke that triathletes possess zero bike handling skills. Here's your chance to prove them wrong. Practice key skills such as gear changes, cornering, hill climbs, and hill descents, and you'll shave valuable seconds off your bike section. You're also much less likely to fall off.

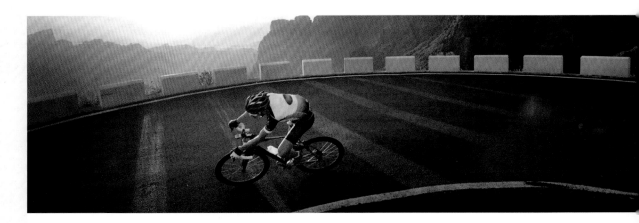

PEDALING

To the beginner, pedaling may seem like a pretty simple action, but there are ways you can make it more efficient, especially if you're using clipless pedals (see page 53) rather than flat pedals.

When pedaling, imagine that the circular motion of each leg is a clock face. To get maximum power out of your pedaling, you need to ensure your foot is driving the pedal all the way round that clock face. From 12 o'clock to 6 o'clock this is obvious since gravity is on your side as you push down. But from 6 o'clock to 12 o'clock, too, you should still be driving by pulling your foot upward. Don't allow your legs to get lazy on any part of each revolution.

And remember that pedaling is a two-leg motion. Think about pulling up with one pedal at the same time as you are pushing down with the other.

And, crucially, if you're using normal flat pedals, always make sure the point of contact between your foot and the pedal is the ball of your foot. If you wrongly use the middle of your foot or your heel, you'll end up pedaling really inefficiently.

CADENCE

This is the number of revolutions your pedals make every minute. As a triathlon beginner, you need to adopt a cadence that your feel comfortable with—not too fast, not too slow. But there will be periods during your training (and during your race) when you increase or decrease your cadence, depending on how strong your legs are, how fit you're feeling, the incline of the road, and which gear you're in, etc. As a general rule, cyclists with more muscly legs but who have less cardiovascular fitness tend to adopt a tougher gear and drive the pedals more slowly; while cyclists with less muscly legs but who have more cardiovascular fitness tend to ride in an easier gear, but drive the pedals more quickly. During training you can work out which cycling style works best for you.

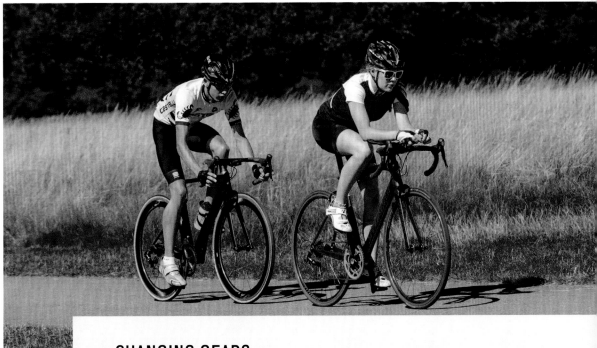

CHANGING GEARS

By the time race day comes around, you should know your bike so well that you can change up and down gears with your eyes closed. Efficient gear changing calls for planning ahead as you need to change gears before the road starts to incline, or before a sharp corner. If you leave it too late, you'll find you lose your momentum. Always change gears smoothly, spinning the pedals softly, not forcefully, as you do so. Don't crunch through the gears as you change them or you'll damage the chain and the teeth of the cogs.

CORNERING

Provided you have the correct tires on your bike, it's highly unlikely your wheels will wash out (i.e. skid away from you) on a corner. But in certain conditions (when it's wet or icy, or there are leaves, sand, or grit on the road), corners can be tricky to negotiate. In a race situation, you want to take the corners as quickly as it's safe to do so, so practice cornering fast during your training. Be well prepared before you reach the corner. Drop down into an easier gear so that you can accelerate once you're through the corner. Stop pedaling and lean your bike into the corner, remembering to keep your inside pedal up, your outside pedal down, with your leg pushing on it. Stay light in your saddle.

If you find you're riding too fast, only brake if you have to. Use mostly the rear brake, and not just the front brake, otherwise you risk your wheel washing out. Head wide into the corner, and then turn tightly, trying to exit the corner from the inside point (the apex). Once you're through the corner, accelerate fast to get back to your previous speed.

HILLS

Get used to including lots of hills in your training rides. Yes, riding uphill hurts, but the more you do it, the less it hurts. See hills as your friends rather than your enemies!

If a hill comes out of nowhere and suddenly gets very steep, you need to change into an easy gear before it starts. If it's a gradual incline, however, slowly change down the gears. Get into the habit of not going too easy too soon. You don't want to be in your easiest gear at the start of the hill since you'll then take longer to ascend it. Once the hill starts to get steep, you can stand out of the saddle to give yourself more drive and more power through the pedals. You'll find it makes the climb easier.

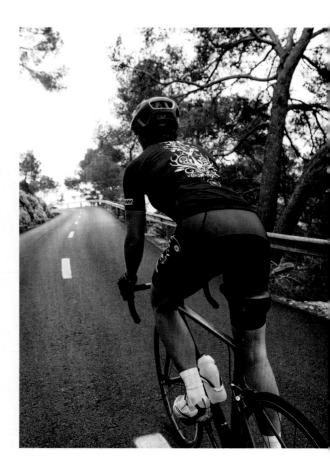

CYCLING DRILLS

Unless you vary your bike training, you'll quickly get bored.
It's not enough simply to head out on the bike for repetitive
road miles. You need to spice things up a bit. How long you
spend on each drill depends on your fitness, and how close
you are to race day. (See Chapter 6: Training Schedules,
pages 90–109.) Always start each drill with at least
10 minutes of easy cycling to warm up.

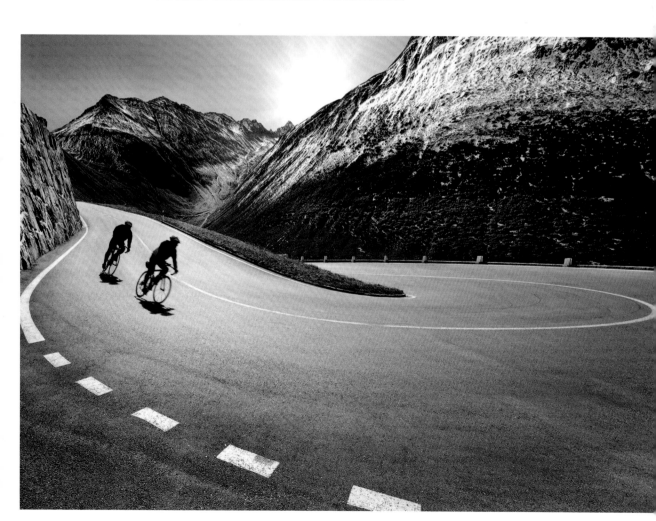

INTERVAL TRAINING

Alternate 5 minutes of medium-paced cycling with 2 minutes of high-paced cycling. Continue alternating at this ratio throughout the drill. This will help you build up your speed on the bike since it gets your heart and other muscles used to pumping really fast. Vary the maximum effort you put in, depending on the incline of the roads you're training on. If you're pushed for time, increase the overall number of minutes you cycle at a high pace, and shorten the sections at a medium pace.

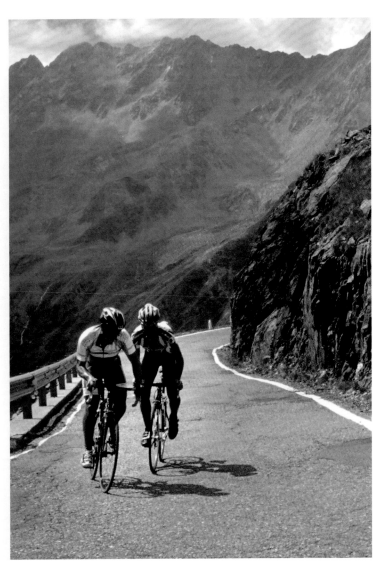

HILL TRAINING

Go training on hilly roads. Mix it up so you get some sections on the flat, some climbing hills, and some descending hills. Even better if some hills are steep and others are less steep. If you live in a very flat region, you'll need to do a stationary bike workout (see page 68) with resistance instead.

ENDURANCE TRAINING

Even if you're doing just a Sprint-distance triathlon, it's a great idea to build some endurance training into your schedule. You can keep the pace medium, but make sure the distance is long. Try to do rides that regularly take you well over an hour. Choose routes with great scenery and varied inclines so you don't get bored.

GROUP TRAINING

If you struggle to fit long rides into a busy schedule of work and/or family life, it's inevitable you'll do a lot of training alone. But you must get used to riding in a pack since this will emulate a race situation. You'll also glean valuable tips from fellow riders.

You might get a group of other triathletes together for a weekend ride or you might join a triathlon or cycling club. It matters not. What matters is that you get used to riding in close proximity to other riders.

Here are some tips for when you're riding in a group:

≡ As a beginner, keep a gap of about a meter between you and the bike in front. Once you gain confidence, you can make this gap shorter.

≡ It's rare that triathletes use their tri bars/aero bars when riding in a tight group because the position of their hands means they can't change direction or brake really quickly. If you do have tri bars, consider dropping a little way behind the group.

≡ Pay attention to the instructions and hand signals from riders in front of you, and pass them on to riders behind you.

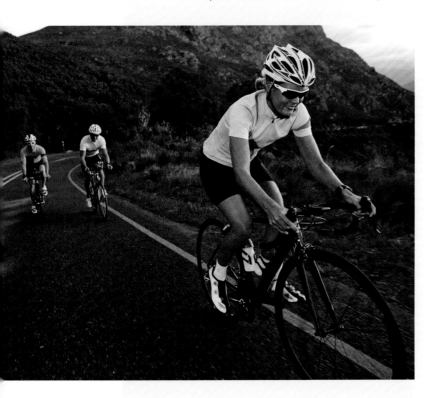

≡ Practice drafting behind other riders. Drafting is when you ride in the slipstream created by the bike in front. In a race situation this allows you to ride just as fast as you normally would, but without expending as much energy. Be aware that in some triathlons bike drafting is legal; in others, it isn't.

≡ If your fellow riders are more experienced than you, ask them lots of questions as you ride. Discuss tactics and equipment from all three disciplines. It's amazing what tips you can pick up.

TURBO TRAINING

In case you're unfamiliar with these devices, a quick note of explanation: turbo trainers let you ride your bike stationary and indoors—perfect for winter training in northern climes. With most models, you suspend your rear wheel in a frame, and cycle as you normally would, pedaling against resistance that you can increase or decrease. Some trainers use magnets to create resistance, some use fluid, some use air, and in others you remove your back wheel and attach your rear forks to it. There are also devices called rollers where you don't remove your back wheel and your bike isn't suspended at all. On these you need to balance as you cycle on the rollers. Come wintertime, when it gets dark, wet, and cold, you'll be spending many long hours grinding out the miles on your turbo trainer.

When using your turbo trainer:

≡ Place it on a smooth, flat surface where you can get a good view of the TV. Let's be honest, long training sessions can be boring, and box sets make the time pass more quickly. Otherwise cue up the stereo with lots of inspirational songs.

≡ You're going to get sweaty, so place a fan in front of you as you ride.

≡ Have a towel handy, too, to wipe away the sweat.

≡ You're going to need at least a couple of water bottles, depending on your workout time.

≡ Use a stopwatch to regulate your turbo sessions. A bike computer is even better.

≡ Always warm up gradually for 10 minutes or so before you start your turbo session.

≡ Sometimes you'll want to smash out some long interval sessions. For these you need to ride at around 70 percent of your maximum heart rate for between 45 minutes and an hour.

≡ Other times you might want to grind out high-intensity sessions. For example, you might alternate 30-second bursts at close to full pace with 2-minute periods at a slow pace.

≡ Always warm down at the end of your session.

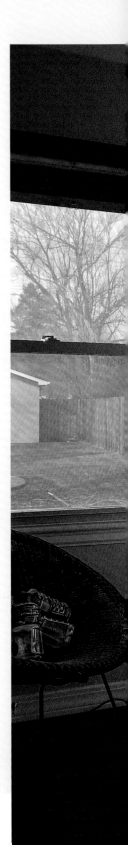

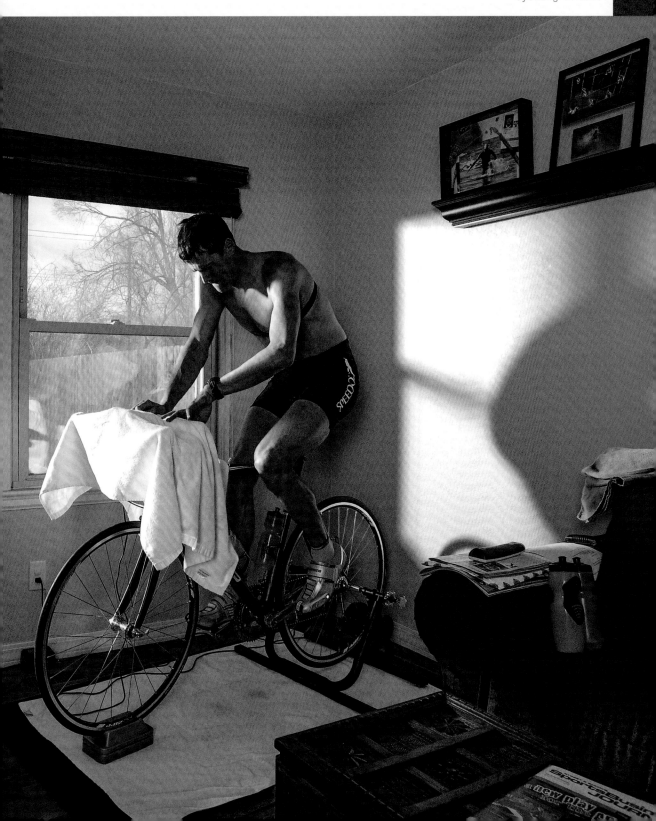

Positive messages

By Luke Tyburski, who completed a 2,000-km triathlon challenge from Morocco to Monaco in 12 days

To keep himself motivated during his long bike-training sessions, Luke Tyburski writes positive messages on a strip of masking tape and then sticks the tape to the headset of his bike. "It might be some motto that inspires me, or names of family I'm close to. When I'm struggling with the bike ride, it really helps." Tyburski also recommends strapping a small (and crucially very light) race mascot to the headset of the bike. It could be a little figurine or a cuddly toy. "Or something that reminds you of tough times you've been through, or of a loved one," he adds. "When you've got your head down and you're focused on clocking up the miles, you'll see it right there in front of your nose."

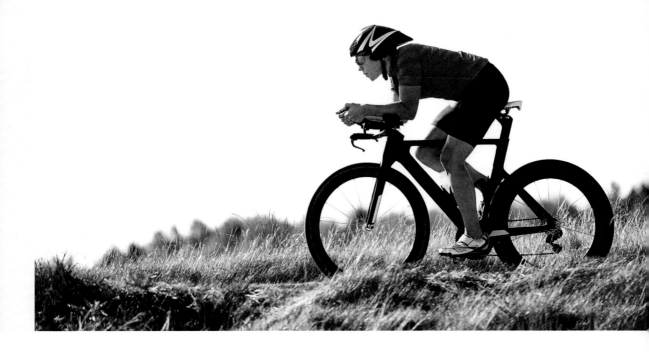

TRIATHLON LEGENDS
Javier Gomez (Spain)

BORN: March 25, 1983, Basel, Switzerland
OLYMPIC GAMES SILVER MEDAL: London 2012
ITU WORLD CHAMPION: 2008, 2010, 2013–2015

For much of his early career Gomez was hampered by a cardiac anomaly, which led sports authorities to ban him from competing for health and safety reasons. But after spending much time and effort in legal courts and medical centers, this Spanish triathlete has proved he has the heart to compete at the very top level. As well as his Olympic silver medal and multiple World Championship titles, he has proved he is excellent at long-course triathlon, too, winning gold in the world's top half Ironman competition (Ironman 70.3 World Championship) and the most demanding off-road triathlon championship (XTERRA World Championship).

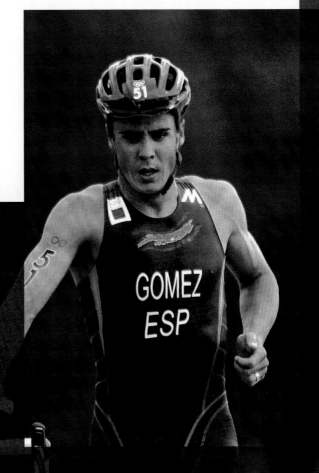

CHAPTER 4

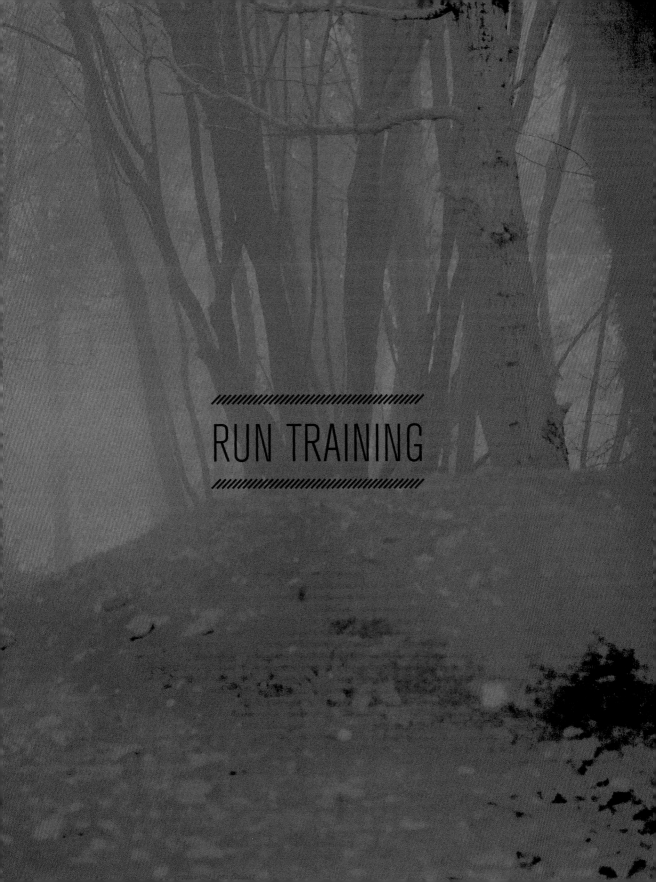

RUN TRAINING

SO WE COME TO THE LAST TRIATHLON DISCIPLINE...

The run is the one that the majority of beginners will find most natural. Everyone can run, even if some people look a bit ungainly. Of the three disciplines it's also the one that's easiest to train for since you can do it any time, anywhere, whatever the weather. But where is the best place to run?

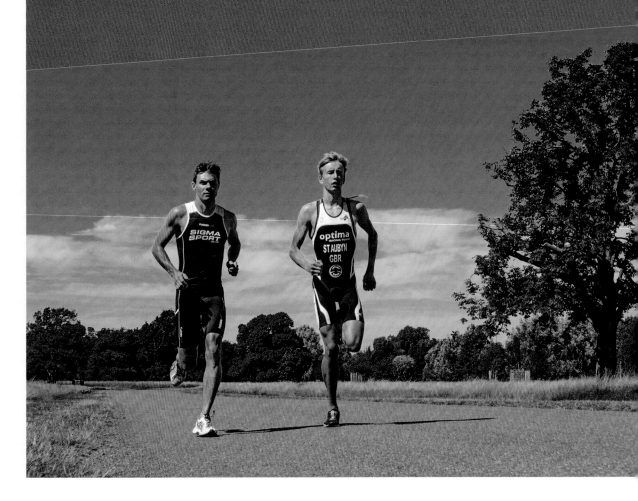

GYM

Running treadmills in the gym are great for when the weather's lousy. They offer good shock absorption, they allow you to monitor your speed and distance accurately, and it's not dangerous to pipe music through your headphones. And, of course, there are no cars in a gym. But let's be honest, gyms are boring. If you're clocking up lots of miles, you need to get outside to break up the monotony. Fresh air and nature will boost you both physiologically and psychologically.

ROAD RUNNING

Most triathlons stage the run section on roads. For that reason you need to get lots of road running under your belt during training. If it's possible (and safe) try to run on asphalt/ tarmac rather than on paving slabs. Asphalt is softer than concrete, therefore sending less impact up through your legs. Over several miles it makes a huge difference. Many city parks offer traffic-calmed roads, which are great for running.

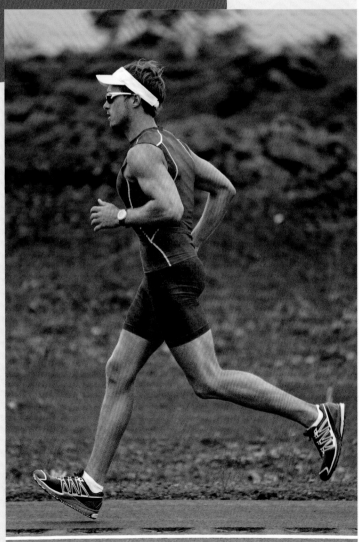

ATHLETICS TRACK

Yes, you can measure your distances accurately on a running track, and the surface reduces the impact in your legs, but given the distance you're training for, an athletics track is fairly dull.

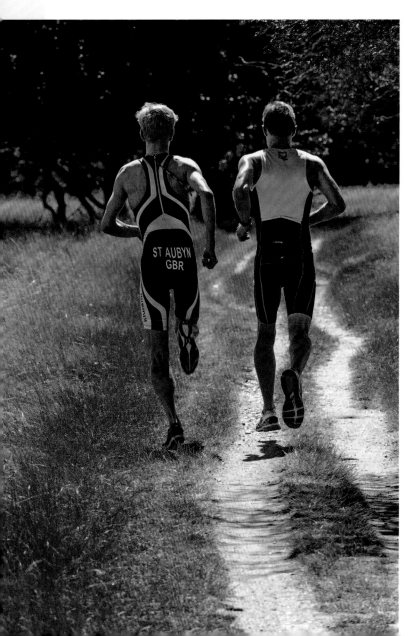

PARK RUNNING

Parks offer a great variety of surfaces: asphalt, dirt trails, grass. There are plenty of other park users and even a bit of nature to distract you from your task.

WOODLAND TRAILS AND COUNTRYSIDE

Just for your own sanity, head out to the countryside and experience running as nature intended. As you engage with nature and enjoy the great outdoors, you'll give yourself a huge mental boost. But be wary of uneven surfaces, especially in the last few weeks leading up to race day. A twisted ankle does not a triathlon win.

RUNNING CLOTHING AND EQUIPMENT

Of the three triathlon disciplines, the run requires the least amount of equipment. Shoes designed specifically for running are obviously crucial, but you can get away with budget clothing. It all depends on how serious you are about your running and whether you plan to train in very cold or very hot weather.

RUNNING SHOES

Peruse your average sports equipment website and you'll be bombarded with hundreds of different brands and models. Lots of choice, yes, but it's confusing. First off you need to decide what surfaces you're likely to be running on. There are shoes designed for road running, off-road shoes designed for trail running, spikes designed for cross-country racing and athletics tracks, barefoot shoes that mimic running barefoot, and racing shoes which are very lightweight. Some brands are now even offering triathlon-specific shoes with elastic laces and an inner lining that doesn't need socks.

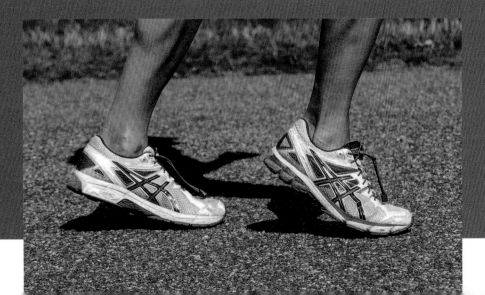

As a beginner, it's best to avoid a specific design of shoe and opt instead for an all-round shoe that will serve you well whether you're running on treadmills, in parks, or on hard surfaces.

Female shoes

No, it's not just marketing and color schemes. The anatomy of a woman's foot is markedly different to a man's. Shoe manufacturers compensate for this in the shoe design.

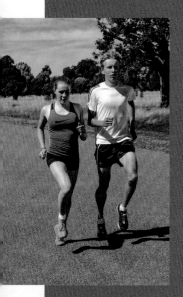

Foot type

Running shoes are designed to compensate for the way your feet pronate—i.e. the way they roll to the side and flatten out as you run. If your foot rolls a lot, you're an over-pronator. If it doesn't roll at all, you're an under-pronator. If you're somewhere in the middle, you have neutral pronation.

There's a way of checking your pronation type. Some people call it the wet foot test:

= Dip your foot in water, shake off the excess water, and then place your foot firmly down on a dry paving slab.

= If you leave a normal footprint, you have neutral pronation and you'll need only a little bit of arch support in your running shoe.

= If you leave a very narrow footprint, then you're an under-pronator with high foot arches, and you'll need cushioned or neutral running shoes with lots of flexibility.

= If you leave a wide footprint, then you're an over-pronator with flatter feet, and you'll need a stability shoe or a shoe with firm support, in order to stop you pronating too much.

Foot strike

Many running shoes offer extra cushioning in the heel. This is great if your style of running is to land heel-first, but if you tend to land with the mid-foot or toe first, then you won't need so much heel cushioning.

Foot size

Always try on running shoes in a store before you buy. (Even if you cheekily end up buying them later online.) Ideally, you should try them on in the middle of the day since your feet are smaller in the mornings and larger in the evenings, after gradually swelling all day. Your toes should have room to wiggle a little bit, but not too much. Remember that different manufacturers offer radically different shoe sizes. Annoyingly, a size 10 in Nike is never quite the same as a size 10 in Adidas.

Stick with your shoe

Once you've found a brand and model that works for you, stick with it. At beginner-level triathlon, you should use the same shoe for training as on race day. Many runners find that if they chop and change between brands and models, they are forced to modify their running style slightly. This can cause injuries.

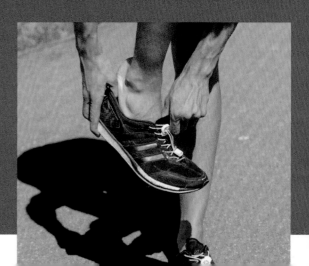

SOCKS

For short runs, normal sports socks are fine, but if you're training over longer distances you may want to invest in double-layer running socks, which help prevent blisters. As you run, the two layers rub against each other, thereby reducing any chafing on the skin of your feet. The socks are often made of wicking material, which draws sweat away from your feet, further reducing the chance of blisters.

SHORTS

Make sure you buy shorts that are specifically designed for running. These normally come with a loose outer layer of wicking material that draws moisture away from your skin as you sweat, plus a tight inner layer that lies next to your skin. That inner layer is crucial, especially for men (for anatomical reasons we don't need to go into here!) It's useful if the shorts have a small zip pocket for your keys or music player.

LEGGINGS

In winter you'll need full-length leggings to keep your leg muscles warm as you run. Again, opt for ones with a useful zip pocket.

JACKET

Running jackets are light, luminous, windproof, and water-resistant. Some pack very tight and can be stored in a small pocket until you need them.

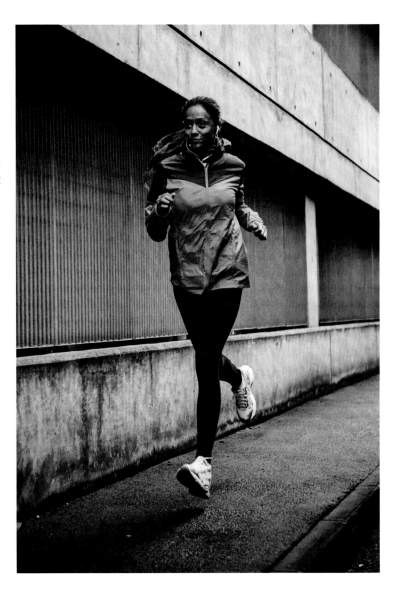

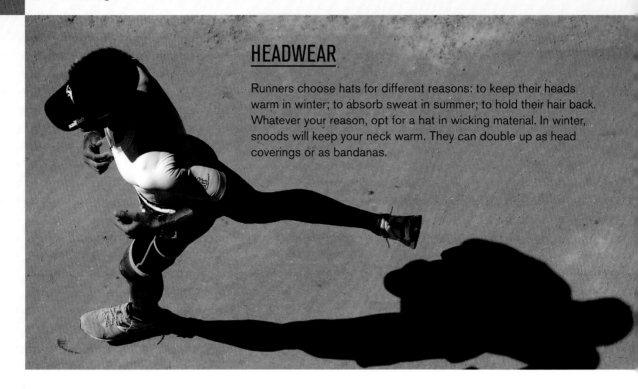

HEADWEAR

Runners choose hats for different reasons: to keep their heads warm in winter; to absorb sweat in summer; to hold their hair back. Whatever your reason, opt for a hat in wicking material. In winter, snoods will keep your neck warm. They can double up as head coverings or as bandanas.

SPORTS BRAS

Women who run without a sports bra risk pain, sagging, and even ligament damage. Most sports bras work by compressing the breasts against your chest, and are supported over the shoulders with wide straps. They cover much of your upper body so that you can run without wearing a T-shirt on top. It's worth buying your sports bra from a specialist running store and having it fitted correctly.

T-SHIRT

Choose an artificial material that wicks away the sweat as you run. Ordinary cotton T-shirts can get wet and heavy as you sweat. For winter training, wear a long-sleeved T-shirt. Choose one in a bright color if you're running near roads.

COMPRESSION CLOTHING

This includes shorts, leggings, and tops that fit tightly against your body, compressing your muscles as you run. You'd normally wear them beneath a looser top layer. The manufacturers of compression clothing boast that it offers all sorts of benefits—it helps your muscles perform better, it helps muscle recovery, it helps you avoid injuries. In truth, different runners report different benefits. At beginner-level triathlon, you've got more important things to worry about than expensive compression clothing. And, yes, it is expensive.

RUNNING TECHNIQUE

Running coaches will bombard you with advice about how to improve your running style. The problem is you've probably adopted a few bad habits. Changing those can risk injury and complicate your training, so if you have a running style that works for you, at beginner-level triathlon at least, you're best advised to stick with it. However, here are a few physiological things to consider.

FOOT STRIKE

Most runners are what are called heel-strikers, in that their feet hit the ground heel-first. A smaller percentage of runners hit the ground with the middle of their feet or their toes first. In recent years there have been various studies claiming that heel-strikers risk injury more than forefoot-strikers. If you're a heel-striker and you find you can train without injury, then stick with your heel-striking style. But it's worth bearing in mind how many extra miles you're going to be running in training. Some experts believe heel-strikers send more impact up through their bodies every time their feet land on the ground, therefore risking injury in the major joints. If you think this is happening with your running, you may want to try adapting your style slightly so that the middle of your foot or your toes strike the ground first. The theory is that this enables your leg muscles to absorb more of the impact on each step, so reducing the impact you send up through the rest of your body.

In general, it's a good idea to step more lightly as you run. Watch professional runners and they seem to almost brush, rather than strike, the ground as they run.

POSTURE

Stay upright, avoid sideways movements, and lean slightly forward as you run. It's important your feet don't land too far forward on each step, otherwise your legs can act as a brake and slow down your pace. Aim to land your feet below your upper body rather than in front of it. Lift your head and look at the ground a few meters ahead of you as you run.

CADENCE

Running cadence is the number of times a minute your feet strike the ground as you run. Try to increase your running cadence slightly so that you reduce the amount of time your feet are in contact with the ground. It will enable you to run more lightly (therefore avoiding injury) and also faster.

KNEE LIFT

Sprinters lift their knees high, but long-distance runners keep their knees lower as they run, thereby saving energy.

ARM MOVEMENT

Sprinters pump their arms like pistons, but for long-distance running you don't want to waste energy. Keep your arm movements small and in a forward direction if you can.

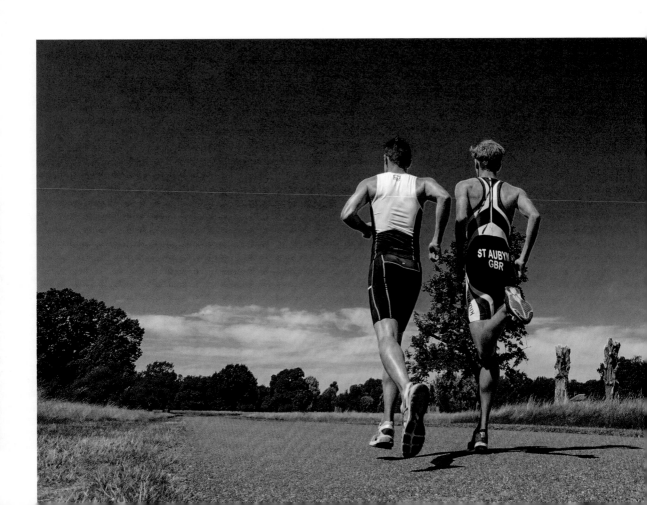

RUNNING DRILLS

Just like in cycling, if you don't vary your running training you'll quickly get bored and uninspired. Running drills can help you work on speed, endurance, and hills, but they also allow you to spice things up a bit. And after lots of miles running round your local park, you're going to need all the spice you can get. How long you spend on each drill depends on your fitness and how close you are to race day. (See Chapter 6: Training Schedules, pages 90–109). Always start each drill with a gentle warm-up run.

INTERVAL RUNNING

It's good to get your body used to running at different speeds. Interval running intersperses fast pace with medium and slow pace. Run for half an hour, with 5-minute slow or medium-paced sections followed by 2-minute fast sections. The fast sections shouldn't be more than about 70 percent of your maximum speed. If you sprint too fast, and you're not used to it, you risk injury.

HILL DRILLS

Most triathlons feature run sections that are fairly flat, but there are occasionally slight inclines, sometimes even medium inclines, during a race, so you need to prepare for these.

Find a hill in a nearby park, or program a hill run into the running treadmill in your gym. A good hill-running drill would be a half-hour normal run with 8–10 short hill sections within it—each around a minute long.

LONG-DISTANCE RUNS

If you're doing a Sprint triathlon, long-distance runs aren't as important. But for an Olympic-distance triathlon, in the latter stages of your training at least, you should be regularly running 10km and longer. The more your body gets used to long distances, the easier you'll find the run section come race day.

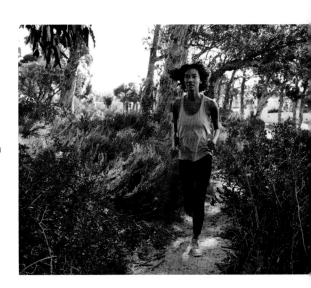

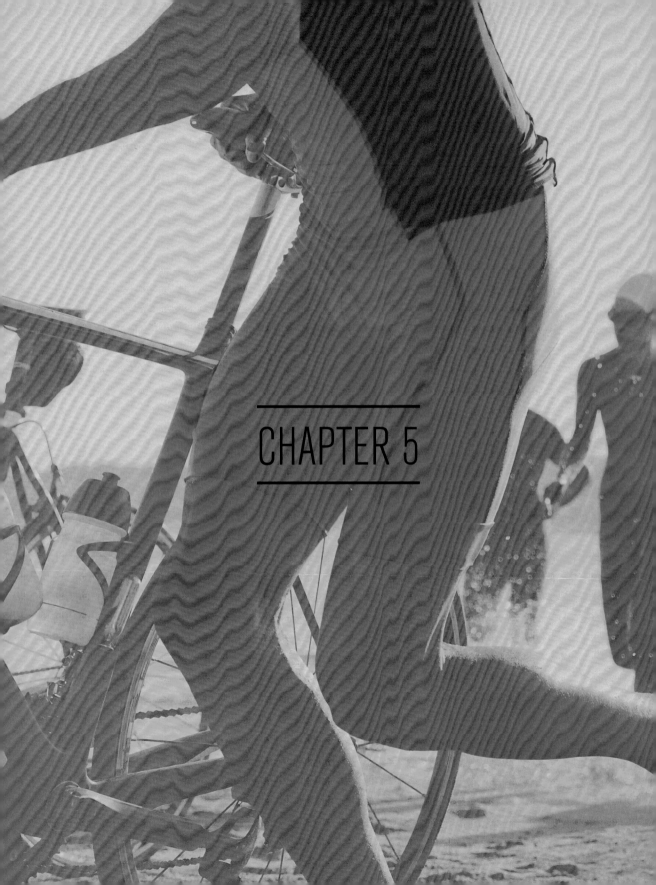

CHAPTER 5

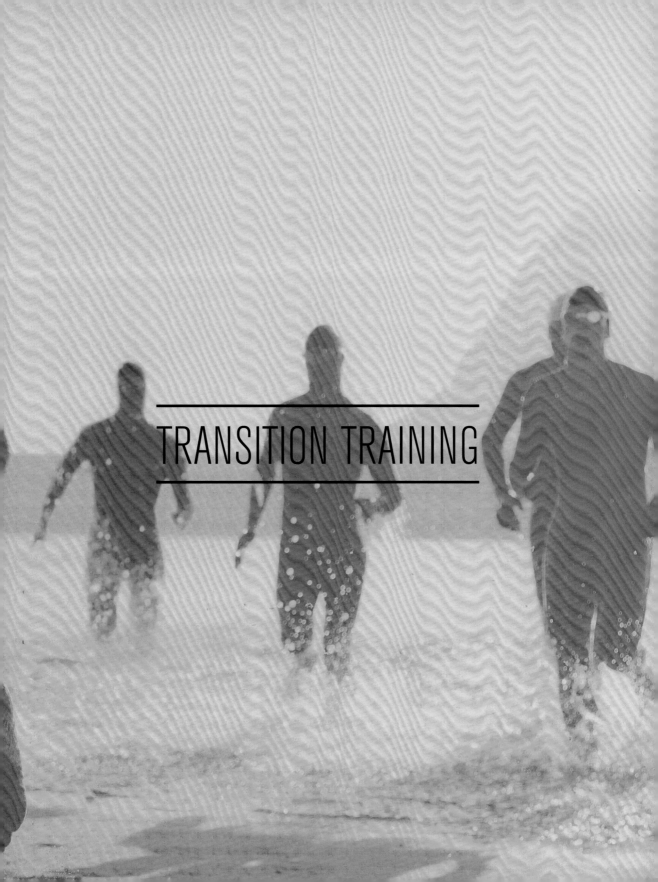

TRANSITION TRAINING

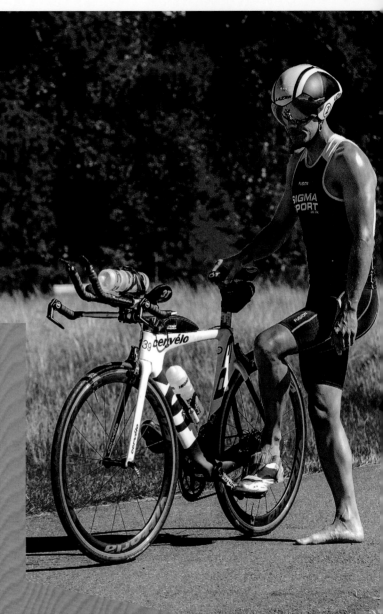

TRIATHLON ISN'T JUST THREE DISCIPLINES.

There's an important fourth discipline: the transitions. There are two transitions: T1 (between the swim section and the bike section) and T2 (between the bike section and the run section). You'll need to practice both of these.

It's good to be aware of what you'll be required to do during the transitions so that you're fully prepared on race day (see pages 122–124 and 128–128). The transition stages include removing your wetsuit quickly (see page 121), strapping on your helmet (you can be penalized or disqualified if you aren't wearing your helmet properly before you exit the transition zone), mounting your bike (see page 124), dismounting your bike (see page 127), and putting your running shoes on (see page 128).

You also need to practice your brick workouts. Bricks are when you combine two disciplines within a single workout, one straight after the other. In triathlon there are two bricks: a swim-to-bike workout and a bike-to-run workout. No one can quite agree on why these workouts are called bricks, but there is a consensus that it's an acronym created from the phrase "bike and run in combination" (BRIC), with a K added on the end. You'll have plenty of time to mull over the veracity of this during the long hours of training.

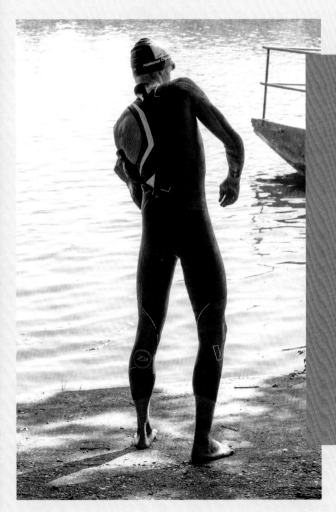

SWIM-TO-BIKE BRICK

Triathletes use their legs as little as possible during the swim section. There's a reason for this: they want to keep their leg muscles fresh for the bike and run sections. Kick too hard in the water and you'll have nothing left in your legs once you mount the bike.

For your swim-bike brick, you don't need to swim and cycle the full distances you normally would during your training schedule. It's the switch between swimming and cycling that you want to get used to. So try to do a workout with three short swims and three short bike rides, so that you get to practice three T1 transitions. A good idea is to do swim sections of 500m followed by 5km bike rides. You can increase these distances as you get fitter.

During the swim section, kick as you normally would during swimming training—i.e. lightly and mainly for balance rather than for propulsion. Then, as you enter the last 50m of your swim, start kicking more vigorously. This will warm up your leg muscles and encourage blood flow to them so that they are ready to start cycling. And remember that, during a race, after exiting the pool or the lake, you will have a short run before you get to your bike. If your legs are cold from the swim, there will be little sensation in your lower legs, and for the first few minutes it can feel very odd. Even more reason to kick your legs vigorously and get the blood flowing during the last 500m of the swim.

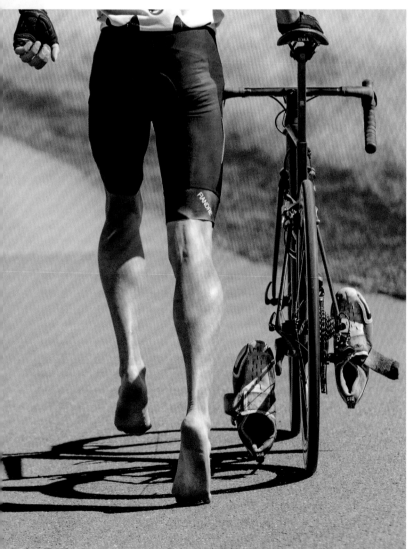

BIKE-TO-RUN BRICK

It can be a very strange sensation switching from cycling to running, since the muscles you use for both disciplines are very different. At the start of the run your legs will feel heavy. Like bricks, in fact. Don't worry—the sensation will pass after you've run a few hundred meters.

Just as in the swim-to-bike brick, for the bike-to-run brick you should try to incorporate three short bike rides and three short runs into your workout, so that you get to practice three T2 transitions. A good idea is to do bike rides of 5km followed by runs of 1.5km. Again, you can increase these distances as you get fitter.

SECURING YOUR BIKE

Here are some ideas:

≡ If your tri suit or wetsuit has a zip pocket, keep your bike key lock in it while you swim.

≡ If you're swim-training in a pool, lock your bike up nearby for a quick transition.

≡ If you're swim-training at a lake, lock your bike up in your car. Keep a change of clothing in the car for the end of your bike ride.

≡ Do your bike-to-run bricks using your own home as the starting and transition point. That way you don't have to worry about bike security.

≡ Do your bricks in the gym. That way you can exit the pool, dry off really quickly, and jump on the stationary bike. A transition from the stationary bike to the running treadmill is even quicker.

≡ Bike-to-run bricks are logistically easier to organize since you aren't dripping wet from the swim.

≡ In very warm weather, there's one really easy way to do a swim-to-bike brick. Cycle down to your local pool and lock your bike up nearby. Leave all your clothing in a small backpack and place it at the end of your pool lane. Once you finish your swim section, exit the pool quickly, put on your shoes and your backpack and immediately jump on your bike and cycle back home. You'll be riding your bike dripping wet so you obviously can't do this in winter.

Pro-Tip

Strange, heavy legs

Enrico Contolini, Colorado-based triathlete and personal trainer

"When you stop biking and start running, the legs feel strange and heavy. The heart rate may go up, as your body tries to switch the blood from flowing into the muscles used for biking to those used for running. This feeling is more pronounced at the start of the run and usually the legs get better as time passes. Brick workouts help shorten the time our legs take to start feeling more normal, thus allowing us to run better and faster. It is not uncommon to experience cramps when starting to run after biking, especially if you're not used to it. As usual, listen to your body and slow down if you feel a cramp coming. A carbohydrate gel and water will also help if you are experiencing cramps due to the decrease in muscle fuel."

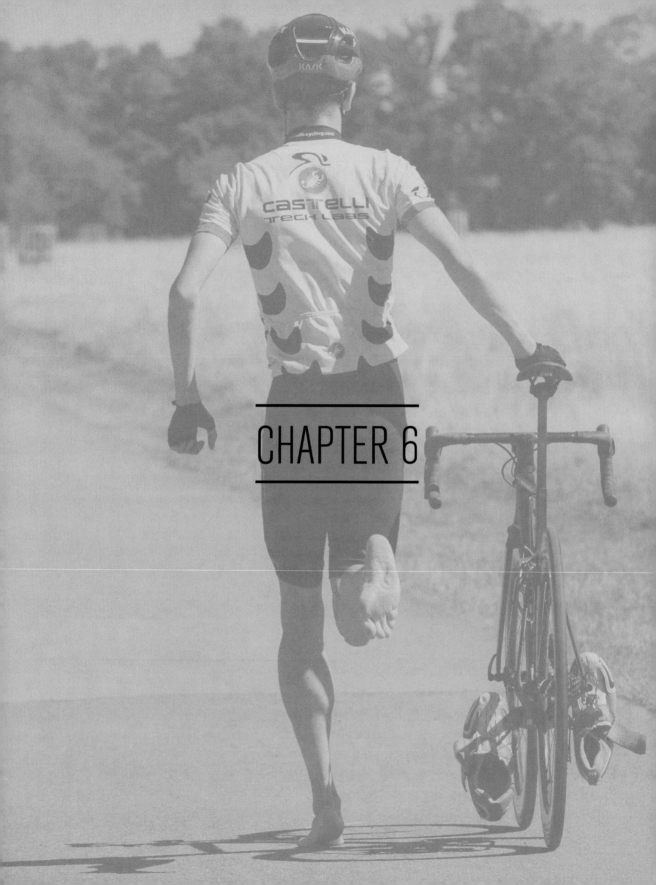

CHAPTER 6

TRAINING SCHEDULES

GIVE YOURSELF A MINIMUM OF THREE MONTHS TO TRAIN FOR YOUR FIRST TRIATHLON.

Whether it's a Sprint distance or an Olympic distance, this amount of training time will ensure you're race-ready and mentally confident. If you already have a good base level of fitness, you can train in a shorter time than this, but there's a chance you'll risk injury by increasing your distances too quickly, or perhaps you'll feel mentally under-prepared.

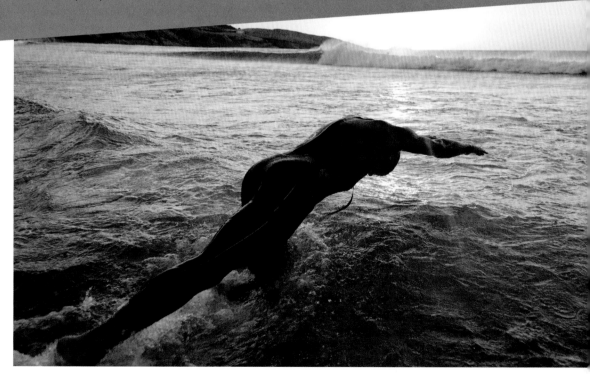

The training schedules in this chapter assume that you're relatively new to all three triathlon disciplines. However, many triathlon debutants are already very strong in one discipline before they approach the sport. If this is the case, you'll find it easy to train longer and harder in that particular discipline than is suggested here. But just because you're a strong cyclist, for example, don't let this be a reason to neglect one of the other disciplines.

Mondays are designated days off. That's because many people with full-time jobs have their trickiest commute on a Monday morning. At weekends they might find it easier to train for longer. Feel free to switch things around so your day off is a different day.

Don't worry if you end up switching disciplines from one day to another. After all, your local pool might not operate lane swimming on certain days; or your bike might end up at the repair shop for a couple of days. You can be flexible. And if you miss a training session altogether, don't beat yourself up. The 12 weeks gives you lots of room to maneuver.

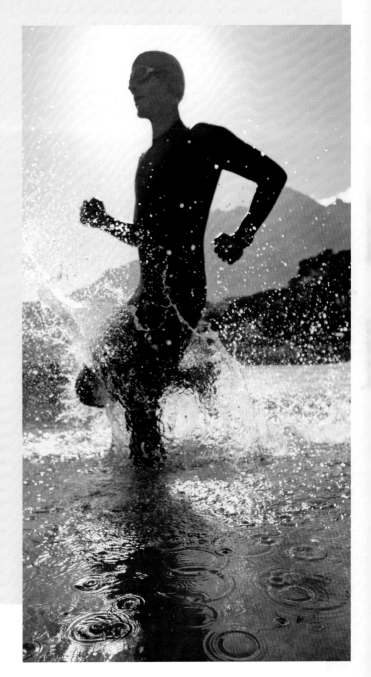

SPRINT TRAINING PLAN

	MONDAY	TUESDAY	WEDNESDAY
WEEK 1	**DAY OFF**	**Swim–300m total** • Warm up–50m easy pace front crawl (or breaststroke if you prefer) • 200m front crawl (or breaststroke if you prefer) at medium pace • Cool down–50m easy breaststroke	**Bike–40 mins total** • Warm up–10 mins at easy pace • 20 mins–medium effort • Cool down–10 mins at easy pace
WEEK 2	**DAY OFF**	**Swim–300m total** • Warm up–50m easy pace front crawl (or breaststroke if you prefer) • 200m front crawl (or breaststroke if you prefer) at medium pace • Cool down–50m easy breaststroke	**Bike–40 mins total** • Warm up–10 mins at easy pace • 20 mins–medium effort • Cool down–10 mins at easy pace
WEEK 3	**DAY OFF**	**Swim–400m total** • Warm up–50m easy pace front crawl • 300m–front crawl at medium pace • Cool down–50m easy pace front crawl	**Bike–50 mins total** • Warm up–10 mins at easy pace • 30 mins–medium effort • Cool down–10 mins at easy pace

THURSDAY	FRIDAY	SATURDAY	SUNDAY
Run–20 mins total • Warm up–5 mins at easy pace • 10 mins–medium effort • Cool down–5 mins at easy pace	**Swim–300m total** • Warm up–50m easy pace front crawl (or breaststroke if you prefer) • 200m front crawl (or breaststroke if you prefer) at medium pace • Cool down–50m easy breaststroke	**Bike–40 mins total** • Warm up–10 mins at easy pace • 20 mins–medium effort • Cool down–10 mins at easy pace	**Run–20 mins total** • Warm up–5 mins at easy pace • 10 mins–medium effort • Cool down–5 mins at easy pace
Run–20 mins total • Warm up–5 mins at easy pace • 10 mins–medium effort • Cool down–5 mins at easy pace	**Swim–300m total** • Warm up–50m easy pace front crawl (or breaststroke if you prefer) • 200m front crawl (or breaststroke if you prefer) at medium pace • Cool down–50m easy breaststroke	**Bike–40 mins total** • Warm up–10 mins at easy pace • 20 mins–medium effort • Cool down–10 mins at easy pace	**Run–20 mins total** • Warm up–5 mins at easy pace • 10 mins–medium effort • Cool down–5 mins at easy pace
Run–30 mins total • Warm up–5 mins at easy pace • 20 mins–medium effort • Cool down–5 mins at easy pace	**Swim–400m total** • Warm up–50m easy pace front crawl • 300m front crawl–medium pace • Cool down–50m easy pace front crawl	**Bike–50 mins total** • Warm up–10 mins at easy pace • 30 mins–medium effort • Cool down–10 mins at easy pace	**Run–30 mins total** • Warm up–5 mins at easy pace • 20 mins–medium effort • Cool down–5 mins at easy pace

	MONDAY	TUESDAY	WEDNESDAY
WEEK 4	**DAY OFF**	**Swim—400m total** • Warm up—50m easy pace front crawl • 300m front crawl—medium pace • Cool down—50m easy pace front crawl	**Bike—50 mins total** • Warm up—10 mins at easy pace • 30 mins—medium effort • Cool down—10 mins at easy pace
WEEK 5	**DAY OFF**	**Swim—600m total** • Warm up—50m easy pace front crawl • 500m front crawl—medium to hard pace • Cool down—50m easy pace front crawl	**Bike—16km total** • Warm up for 2km—easy pace • 12km—medium to hard effort, incorporating some gentle hills • Cool down—2km at easy pace
WEEK 6	**DAY OFF**	**Swim—600m total** • Warm up—50m easy pace front crawl • 500m front crawl—medium to hard pace • Cool down—50m easy pace front crawl	**Bike—16km total** • Warm up for 2km—easy pace • 12km—medium to hard effort, incorporating some gentle hills • Cool down—2km at easy pace

THURSDAY	FRIDAY	SATURDAY	SUNDAY
Run—30 mins total	**Swim—400m total**	**Bike—50 mins total**	**Run—30 mins total**
• Warm up—5 mins at easy pace • 20 mins—medium effort • Cool down—5 mins at easy pace	• Warm up—50m easy pace front crawl • 300m front crawl— medium pace • Cool down—50m easy pace front crawl	• Warm up—10 mins at easy pace • 30 mins—medium effort • Cool down—10 mins at easy pace	• Warm up—5 mins at easy pace • 20 mins—medium effort • Cool down—5 mins at easy pace
Run—5km total	**Swim—600m total**	**Bike—16km total**	**Run—5km total**
• Warm up for 1km— easy pace • 3km—medium to hard effort • Cool down for 1km— easy pace	• Warm up—50m easy pace front crawl • 500m front crawl— medium to hard pace • Cool down—50m easy pace front crawl	• Warm up for 2km— easy pace • 12km—medium to hard effort, incorporating some gentle hills • Cool down—2km at easy pace	• Warm up for 1km— easy pace • 3km—medium to hard effort • Cool down for 1km— easy pace
Run—5km total	**Swim—600m total**	**Bike—16km total**	**Run—5km total**
• Warm up for 1km— easy pace • 3km— medium to hard effort • Cool down for 1km— easy pace	• Warm up—50m easy pace front crawl • 500m front crawl— medium to hard pace • Cool down—50m easy pace front crawl	• Warm up for 2km— easy pace • 12km—medium to hard effort, incorporating some gentle hills • Cool down—2km at easy pace	• Warm up for 1km— easy pace • 3km—medium to hard effort • Cool down for 1km— easy pace

	MONDAY	TUESDAY	WEDNESDAY
WEEK 7	**DAY OFF**	**Swim—700m total** • Warm up—50m easy pace front crawl • 600m front crawl—medium to hard pace • Cool down—50m easy pace front crawl	**Bike—20km total** • Warm up for 2km—easy pace • 16km—medium to hard effort, incorporating some gentle hills • Cool down for 2km—easy pace
WEEK 8	**DAY OFF**	**Interval swimming—600m total** • Warm up—50m easy pace front crawl • Swim 10 x 50m—hard pace with 1 minute's rest between each 50m section • Cool down—50m easy pace front crawl	**Interval biking—16km total** • Warm up for 2km—easy pace • Bike 8 x 1km at hard pace, with 500m freewheeling in between each 1km section • Cool down—2km at easy pace
WEEK 9	**DAY OFF**	**Swim—850m total** • Warm up—50m easy pace front crawl • 750m front crawl—medium to hard pace (this is your race distance) • Cool down—50m easy pace front crawl	**Bike—20km total** • Warm up for 2km—easy pace • 16km—medium to hard effort, incorporating some gentle hills • Cool down—2km at easy pace

THURSDAY	FRIDAY	SATURDAY	SUNDAY
Run—5km total • Warm up for 1km—easy pace • 3km—medium to hard effort • Cool down for 1km—easy pace	**Swim—700m total** • Warm up—50m easy pace front crawl • 600m front crawl—medium to hard pace • Cool down—50m easy pace front crawl	**Bike—20km total** • Warm up for 2km—easy pace • 16km—medium to hard effort, incorporating some gentle hills • Cool down for 2km—easy pace	**Run—5km total** • Warm up for 1km—easy pace • 3km—medium to hard effort • Cool down for 1km—easy pace
Interval running—5km total • Warm up for 1km—easy pace • Run 10 x 300m—medium to hard pace with 1 minute's rest between each 300m section • Cool down for 1km—easy pace	**Interval swimming—600m total** • Warm up—50m easy pace front crawl • Swim 10 x 50m—hard pace with 1 minute's rest between each 50m section • Cool down—50m easy pace front crawl	**Interval biking—16km total** • Warm up for 2km—easy pace • Bike 8 x 1km at hard pace, with 500m freewheeling in between each 1km section • Cool down—2km at easy pace	**Brick (bike to run)—bike 10km, then run 5km** • Warm up for 2km on the bike • Ride 8km—medium to hard effort on the bike • Transition quickly to the run • Warm-up run for 1km • Run—3km at medium effort • Cool-down run for 1km
Run—7km total • Warm up for 1km—easy pace • 5km—medium to hard effort • Cool down for 1km—easy pace	**Swim—850m total** • Warm up—50m easy pace front crawl • 750m front crawl—medium to hard pace (this is your race distance) • Cool down—50m easy pace front crawl	**Bike—20km total** • Warm up for 2km—easy pace • 16km—medium to hard effort, incorporating some gentle hills • Cool down—2km at easy pace	**Brick (bike to run)—bike 20km, then run 5km** • Warm up for 2km on the bike • Ride 18km—medium to hard effort on the bike • Transition quickly to the run • Warm-up run for 1km • Run 3km—medium effort • Cool-down run for 1km

	MONDAY	TUESDAY	WEDNESDAY
WEEK 10	**DAY OFF**	**Swim—850m total** • Warm up—50m easy pace front crawl • 750m front crawl—medium to hard pace (this is your race distance) • Cool down—50m easy pace front crawl	**Brick (bike to run)—bike 20km, then run 5km** • Warm up for 2km on the bike • Ride 18km—medium to hard effort on the bike • Transition quickly to the run • Warm-up run for 1km • Run 3km—medium effort • Cool-down run for 1km
WEEK 11	**DAY OFF**	**Swim—400m total** • Warm up—50m easy pace front crawl • 300m front crawl—medium pace • Cool down—50m easy pace front crawl	**Brick (bike to run)—bike 15km, then run 3km** • Warm up for 2km on the bike • Ride 13km—medium to hard effort on the bike • Transition quickly to the run • Warm-up run for 1km • Run 1km—medium effort • Cool-down run for 1km
WEEK 12	**DAY OFF**	**Swim—300m total** • Warm up—50m easy pace front crawl • 200m front crawl—medium pace • Cool down—50m easy pace front crawl	**Brick (bike to run)—bike 10km, then run 3km** • Warm up for 2km on the bike • Ride 8km—medium effort on the bike • Transition quickly to the run • Warm-up run for 1km • Run 1km—medium effort • Cool-down run for 1km

THURSDAY	FRIDAY	SATURDAY	SUNDAY
Run–5km total • Warm up for 1km—easy pace • 3km—medium to hard effort • Cool down for 1km—easy pace	**Swim–850m total** • Warm up—50m easy pace front crawl • 750m front crawl—medium to hard pace (this is your race distance) • Cool down—50m easy pace front crawl	**Bike–20km total** • Warm up for 2km—easy pace • 16km—medium to hard effort, incorporating some gentle hills • Cool down—2km at easy pace	**Brick (bike to run)–bike 20km, then run 5km** • Warm up for 2km on the bike • Ride 18km—medium to hard effort on the bike • Transition quickly to the run • Warm-up run for 1km • Run 3km—medium effort • Cool-down run for 1km
Run–20 mins total • Warm up–5 mins at easy pace • 10 mins—medium effort • Cool down for 5 mins—easy pace	**Swim–400m total** • Warm up–50m easy pace front crawl • 300m front crawl—medium pace • Cool down—50m easy pace front crawl	**Bike–40 mins total** • Warm up 10 mins—easy pace • 20 mins—medium effort • Cool down 10 mins—easy pace	**Brick (bike to run)–bike 15km, then run 3km** • Warm up for 2km on the bike • Ride 13km—medium to hard effort on the bike • Transition quickly to the run • Warm-up run for 1km • Run 1km—medium effort • Cool-down run for 1km
DAY OFF	**Swim–300m total** • Warm up—50m easy pace front crawl • 200m front crawl—medium pace • Cool down—50m easy pace front crawl	**Brick (bike to run)–bike 10km, then run 3km** • Warm up for 2km on the bike • Ride 8km—medium effort on the bike • Transition quickly to the run • Warm-up run for 1km • Run 1km—medium effort • Cool-down run for 1km	**RACE DAY**

OLYMPIC TRAINING PLAN

	MONDAY	TUESDAY	WEDNESDAY
WEEK 1	**DAY OFF**	**Swim–300m total** • Warm up–50m easy pace front crawl (or breaststroke if you prefer) • 200m front crawl (or breaststroke if you prefer) at medium pace • Cool down–50m easy breaststroke	**Bike–40 mins total** • Warm up–10 mins at easy pace • 20 mins–medium effort • Cool down–10 mins at easy pace
WEEK 2	**DAY OFF**	**Swim–300m total** • Warm up–50m easy pace front crawl (or breaststroke if you prefer) • 200m front crawl (or breaststroke if you prefer) at medium pace • Cool down–50m easy breaststroke	**Bike–40 mins total** • Warm up–10 mins at easy pace • 20 mins–medium effort • Cool down–10 mins at easy pace
WEEK 3	**DAY OFF**	**Swim–400m total** • Warm up–50m easy pace front crawl • 300m–front crawl at medium pace • Cool down–50m easy pace front crawl	**Bike–50 mins total** • Warm up–10 mins at easy pace • 30 mins–medium effort • Cool down–10 mins at easy pace

THURSDAY	FRIDAY	SATURDAY	SUNDAY
Run–20 mins total • Warm up–5 mins at easy pace • 10 mins–medium effort • Cool down–5 mins at easy pace	**Swim–300m total** • Warm up–50m easy pace front crawl (or breaststroke if you prefer) • 200m front crawl (or breaststroke if you prefer) at medium pace • Cool down–50m easy breaststroke	**Bike–40 mins total** • Warm up–10 mins at easy pace • 20 mins–medium effort • Cool down–10 mins at easy pace	**Run–20 mins total** • Warm up–5 mins at easy pace • 10 mins–medium effort • Cool down–5 mins at easy pace
Run–20 mins total • Warm up–5 mins at easy pace • 10 mins–medium effort • Cool down–5 mins at easy pace	**Swim–300m total** • Warm up–50m easy pace front crawl (or breaststroke if you prefer) • 200m front crawl (or breaststroke if you prefer) at medium pace • Cool down–50m easy breaststroke	**Bike–40 mins total** • Warm up–10 mins at easy pace • 20 mins–medium effort • Cool down–10 mins at easy pace	**Run–20 mins total** • Warm up–5 mins at easy pace • 10 mins–medium effort • Cool down–5 mins at easy pace
Run–30 mins total • Warm up–5 mins at easy pace • 20 mins–medium effort • Cool down–5 mins at easy pace	**Swim–400m total** • Warm up–50m easy pace front crawl • 300m front crawl–medium pace • Cool down–50m easy pace front crawl	**Bike–50 mins total** • Warm up–10 mins at easy pace • 30 mins–medium effort • Cool down–10 mins at easy pace	**Run–30 mins total** • Warm up–5 mins at easy pace • 20 mins–medium effort • Cool down–5 mins at easy pace

	MONDAY	TUESDAY	WEDNESDAY
WEEK 4	**DAY OFF**	**Swim–500m total** • Warm up–50m easy pace front crawl • 400m front crawl–medium pace • Cool down–50m easy pace front crawl	**Bike–50 mins total** • Warm up–10 mins at easy pace • 30 mins–medium effort • Cool down–10 mins at easy pace
WEEK 5	**DAY OFF**	**Swim–600m total** • Warm up–50m easy pace front crawl • 500m front crawl–medium to hard pace • Cool down–50m easy pace front crawl	**Bike–16km total** • Warm up for 2km–easy pace • 12km–medium to hard effort, incorporating some gentle hills • Cool down–2km at easy pace
WEEK 6	**DAY OFF**	**Swim–800m total** • Warm up–50m easy pace front crawl • 700m front crawl–medium to hard pace • Cool down–50m easy pace front crawl	**Bike–20km total** • Warm up for 2km–easy pace • 16km–medium to hard effort, incorporating some gentle hills • Cool down–2km at easy pace

THURSDAY	FRIDAY	SATURDAY	SUNDAY
Run–30 mins total • Warm up–5 mins at easy pace • 20 mins–medium effort • Cool down–5 mins at easy pace	**Swim–500m total** • Warm up–50m easy pace front crawl • 400m front crawl–medium pace • Cool down–50m easy pace front crawl	**Bike–50 mins total** • Warm up–10 mins at easy pace • 30 mins–medium effort • Cool down–10 mins at easy pace	**Run–30 mins total** • Warm up–5 mins at easy pace • 20 mins–medium effort • Cool down–5 mins at easy pace
Run–5km total • Warm up for 1km–easy pace • 3km–medium to hard effort • Cool down for 1km–easy pace	**Swim–600m total** • Warm up–50m easy pace front crawl • 500m front crawl–medium to hard pace • Cool down–50m easy pace front crawl	**Bike–16km total** • Warm up for 2km–easy pace • 12km–medium to hard effort, incorporating some gentle hills • Cool down–2km at easy pace	**Run–5km total** • Warm up for 1km–easy pace • 3km–medium to hard effort • Cool down for 1km–easy pace
Run–7km total • Warm up for 1km–easy pace • 5km–medium to hard effort • Cool down for 1km–easy pace	**Swim–800m total** • Warm up–50m easy pace front crawl • 700m front crawl–medium to hard pace • Cool down–50m easy pace front crawl	**Bike–20km total** • Warm up for 2km–easy pace • 16km–medium to hard effort, incorporating some gentle hills • Cool down–2km at easy pace	**Run–7km total** • Warm up for 1km–easy pace • 5km–medium to hard effort • Cool down for 1km–easy pace

	MONDAY	TUESDAY	WEDNESDAY
WEEK 7	**DAY OFF**	**Swim–1km total** • Warm up—50m easy pace front crawl • 900m front crawl—medium to hard pace • Cool down—50m easy pace front crawl	**Bike–30km total** • Warm up—2km at easy pace • 26km—medium to hard effort, incorporating some gentle hills • Cool down—2km at easy pace
WEEK 8	**DAY OFF**	**Interval swimming–700m total** • Warm up—50m easy pace front crawl • Swim 12 x 50m—hard pace with 1 minute's rest between each 50m section • Cool down—50m easy pace front crawl	**Interval biking–20km total** • Warm up for 2km—easy pace • Bike 11 x 1km—hard pace, with 500m freewheeling in between each 1km section • Cool down—2km at easy pace
WEEK 9	**DAY OFF**	**Swim–1.6km total** • Warm up—50m easy pace front crawl • 1.5km front crawl—medium to hard pace (this is your race distance) • Cool down—50m easy pace front crawl	**Bike–40km total** • Warm up for 2km—easy pace • 36km—medium to hard effort, incorporating some gentle hills • Cool down—2km at easy pace

THURSDAY	FRIDAY	SATURDAY	SUNDAY
Run–8km total • Warm up for 1km—easy pace • 6km—medium to hard effort • Cool down for 1km—easy pace	**Swim–1km total** • Warm up—50m easy pace front crawl • 900m front crawl—medium to hard pace • Cool down—50m easy pace front crawl	**Bike–30km total** • Warm up—2km at easy pace • 26km—medium to hard effort, incorporating some gentle hills • Cool down—2km at easy pace	**Run–8km total** • Warm up for 1km—easy pace • 6km—medium to hard effort • Cool down for 1km—easy pace
Interval running–5km total • Warm up for 1km—easy pace • Run 10 x 300m—medium to hard pace with 1 minute's rest between each 300m section • Cool down for 1km—easy pace	**Interval swimming–700m total** • Warm up—50m easy pace front crawl • Swim 12 x 50m—hard pace with 1 minute's rest between each 50m section • Cool down—50m easy pace front crawl	**Interval biking–20km total** • Warm up for 2km—easy pace • Bike 11 x 1km—hard pace, with 500m freewheeling in between each 1km section • Cool down—2km at easy pace	**Brick (bike to run)–bike 20km, then run 8km** • Warm up for 2km on the bike • Ride 18km—medium to hard effort on the bike • Transition quickly to the run • Warm-up run for 1km • Run 6km—medium effort • Cool-down run for 1km
Run–10km total • Warm up for 1km—easy pace • 8km—medium to hard effort • Cool down for 1km—easy pace	**Swim–1.6km total** • Warm up—50m easy pace front crawl • 1.5km front crawl—medium to hard pace (this is your race distance) • Cool down—50m easy pace front crawl	**Bike–40km total** • Warm up for 2km—easy pace • 36km—medium to hard effort, incorporating some gentle hills • Cool down—2km at easy pace	**Brick (bike to run)–bike 30km, then run 8km** • Warm up for 2km on the bike • Ride 28km—medium to hard effort on the bike • Transition quickly to the run • Warm-up run for 1km • Run 6km—medium effort • Cool-down run for 1km

	MONDAY	TUESDAY	WEDNESDAY
WEEK 10	**DAY OFF**	**Swim—1.6km total** • Warm up—50m easy pace front crawl • 1.5km front crawl—medium to hard pace (this is your race distance) • Cool down—50m easy pace front crawl	**Brick (bike to run)—bike 30km, then run 8km** • Warm up for 2km on the bike • Ride 28km—medium to hard effort on the bike • Transition quickly to the run • Warm-up run for 1km • Run 6km—medium effort • Cool-down run for 1km
WEEK 11	**DAY OFF**	**Swim—800m total** • Warm up—50m easy pace front crawl • 700m front crawl—medium pace • Cool down—50m easy pace front crawl	**Brick (bike to run)—bike 20km, then run 8km** • Warm up for 2km on the bike • Ride 18km—medium to hard effort on the bike • Transition quickly to the run • Warm-up run for 1km • Run 6km—medium effort • Cool-down run for 1km
WEEK 12	**DAY OFF**	**Swim—400m total** • Warm up—50m easy pace front crawl • 300m front crawl—medium pace • Cool down—50m easy pace front crawl	**Brick (bike to run)—bike 20km, then run 5km** • Warm up for 2km on the bike • Ride 18km—medium to hard effort on the bike • Transition quickly to the run • Warm-up run for 1km • Run 3km—medium effort • Cool-down run for 1km

THURSDAY	FRIDAY	SATURDAY	SUNDAY
Run—10km total	**Swim—1.6km total**	**Bike—40km total**	**Brick (bike to run)—bike 30km, then run 8km**
• Warm up for 1km— easy pace	• Warm up—50m easy pace front crawl	• Warm up for 2km— easy pace	• Warm up for 2km on the bike
• 8km—medium to hard effort	• 1.5km front crawl— medium to hard pace (this is your race distance)	• 36km—medium to hard effort, incorporating some gentle hills	• Ride 28km—medium to hard effort on the bike
• Cool down for 1km— easy pace	• Cool down—50m easy pace front crawl	• Cool down—2km at easy pace	• Transition quickly to the run
			• Warm-up run for 1km
			• Run 6km—medium effort
			• Cool-down run for 1km
Run—7km total	**Swim—800m total**	**Bike—20km total**	**Brick (bike to run)—bike 20km, then run 8km**
• Warm up for 1km— easy pace	• Warm up—50m easy pace front crawl	• Warm up for 2km— easy pace	• Warm up for 2km on the bike
• 5km—medium to hard effort	• 700m front crawl— medium pace	• 16km—medium to hard effort, incorporating some gentle hills	• Ride 18km—medium to hard effort on the bike
• Cool down for 1km— easy pace	• Cool down—50m easy pace front crawl	• Cool down—2km at easy pace	• Transition quickly to the run
			• Warm-up run for 1km
			• Run 6km—medium effort
			• Cool-down run for 1km
DAY OFF	**Brick (bike to run)— bike 20km, then run 5km**	**Swim—400m total**	**RACE DAY**
	• Warm up for 2km on the bike	• Warm up—50m easy pace front crawl	
	• Ride 18km—medium to hard effort on the bike	• 300m front crawl— medium pace	
	• Transition quickly to the run	• Cool down—50m easy pace front crawl	
	• Warm-up run for 1km		
	• Run 3km—medium effort		
	• Cool-down run for 1km		

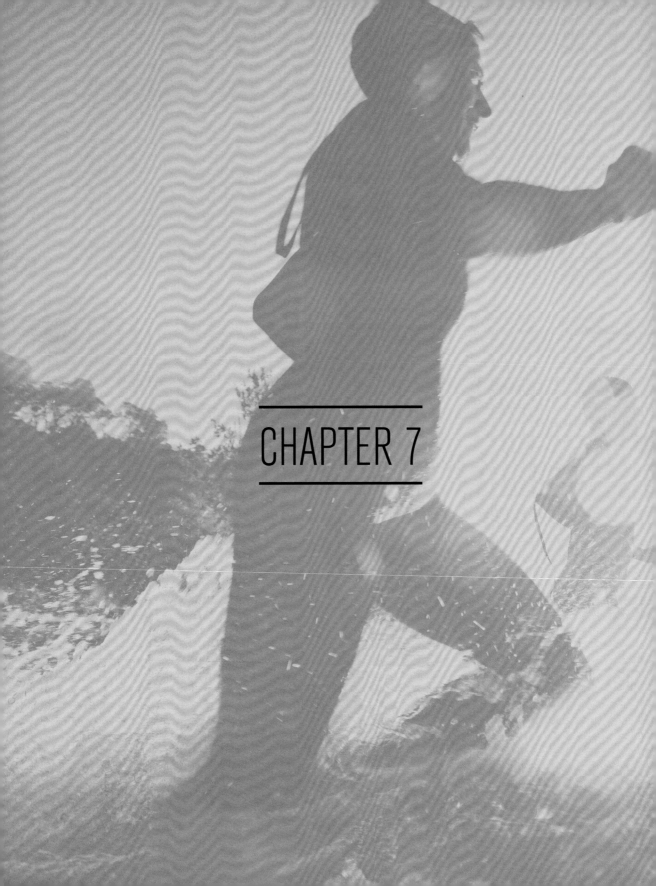

CHAPTER 7

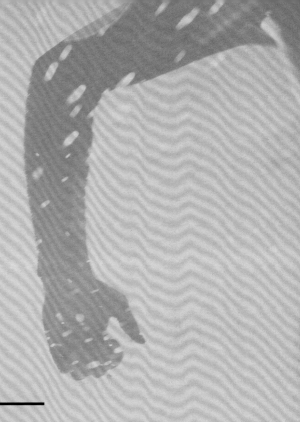

RACE DAY

THE BIG DAY HAS ARRIVED.

This is why you've been doing all your hours of training. You're fit, you're mentally prepared, you're confident, and, God knows, you're definitely going to complete your triathlon race. Talking of God, don't worry if you didn't stick religiously to your training schedule. After all, it's only a Sprint or Olympic distance that you're facing, right? You're not doing an Ironman. And your aim isn't to win—just to finish and have fun in the process.

Triathlon isn't a complicated sport, but thanks to the three different disciplines (four, if you count transitions), there will be more than a few hiccups along the way. The following race tips will arm you with all the knowledge you need to smooth out those hiccups wherever possible.

THE NIGHT BEFORE

Before the race you will be supplied with a no doubt lengthy list of rules. Few people bother reading them and then, come race day, they suddenly realize they're wearing their race number in the wrong place, or they're unsure which exit to take on the final lap of the run. Be the competitor who *does* read the race rules. It will give you extra confidence.

A good night's sleep will put you in good stead for your race. It's important to eat well, especially carbohydrates (see page 20) and drink lots of water the day before your race to ensure you're properly hydrated.

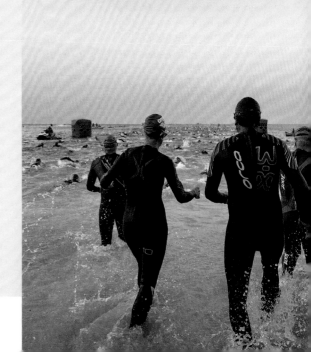

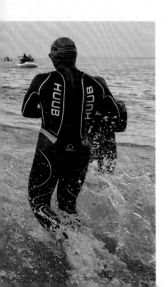

PREPARING YOUR KIT

Lay out all your kit the day before to check you have what you need. You'll just want to grab and go on the morning of the triathlon itself.

GENERAL
- Race details
- Race number (supplied by the race organizer)
- Race timing chip (supplied by the race organizer)
- Watch
- Sunscreen
- Race belt
- Transition towel
- Race food and drink

SWIMMING GEAR
- Tri suit (or swimming trunks/ swimsuit if you choose not to wear a tri suit)
- Wetsuit
- Wetsuit lubricant
- Goggles
- Anti-fogging spray (optional)
- Swimming hat (often supplied by the race organizer)

BIKE GEAR
- Bike
- Helmet
- Cycling glasses
- Cycling shoes
- Cycling shorts and jersey (if you're not wearing a tri suit)
- Bike pump
- Spare inner tubes
- Tire levers and tools
- Water bottle(s)

RUNNING GEAR
- Running shorts and shirt (if you're not wearing a tri suit)
- Running shoes
- Socks
- Hat

TIMING CHIP
Most race organizers require you to wear a race timing chip on your ankle throughout the race. Make sure it's securely attached to your ankle—the left ankle, so there's no risk of it catching on the bike chain ring as you pedal.

THE MORNING OF THE RACE

Eat breakfast at least two hours before the race is due to start to give you time to digest it, and to provide the fuel you need.

Try to recce the course of the triathlon as much as you can. Pay particular attention to the entry and exit of the swim, and the transition areas. The fewer surprises, the better.

About 20 minutes before the start of the race do some warm-up exercises or a gentle jog. But keep it gentle. Nothing too strenuous.

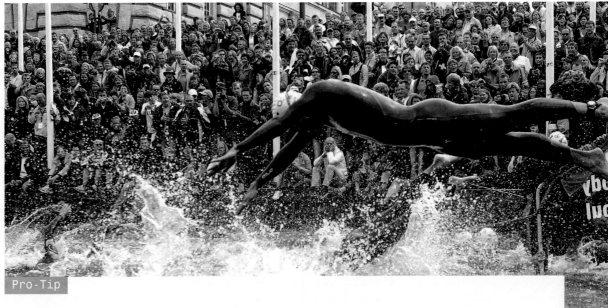

Pro-Tip

Pre-race food

Alistair Brownlee, Olympic triathlon gold medalist

"I can eat two hours before a race, but some people need longer to digest—maybe three or even four hours. You should have tried out what's best for your body well before race day. Don't eat anything too complicated. Pasta, a sandwich, any kind of food you digest easily are good. When it comes to hydration, drink a product you've used before. Don't try anything new on race day. People say it's good to drink a Coke after a training swim in open water because it kills any bacteria. But don't drink it when you're actually racing."

TRIATHLON LEGENDS
Paula Newby-Fraser (USA)

BORN: June 2, 1962, Harare, Zimbabwe

IRONMAN WORLD CHAMPION: 1986, 1988, 1989, 1991–1994, 1996

To win the Ironman World Championship once is impressive enough. To win it eight times, as Paula Newby-Fraser has done, might be considered superhuman. No wonder this Zimbabwean-turned-American is considered one of the greatest triathletes of all time.

Newby-Fraser was born in the then Rhodesian capital Harare and brought up in South Africa. Until the early 1990s when she switched allegiance to the USA, she always used to compete under her native Zimbabwe flag. Will anyone ever beat her Ironman World Championship record? It's possible but highly unlikely.

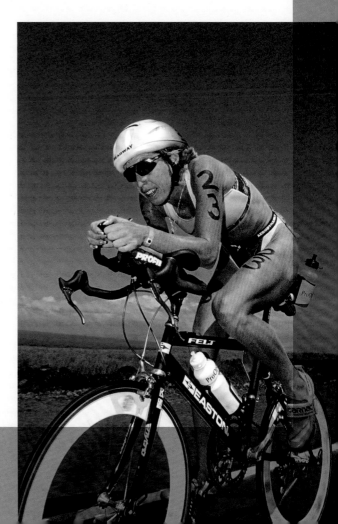

SWIMMING RACING TIPS

Beginners often find the swim section of the race the most daunting. Certainly, if you're facing an open-water swim, those long minutes you wait at the start of the race can be intimidating. While you wait, stand at the back of the field. As a beginner, remember your job is simply to complete this triathlon. Let the other racers scramble for pole position, while you relax at the back of the starting line-up.

≡ Be ready at the start of the swim a minimum of 15 minutes before the starting gun. Remember to wear your tri suit (or your swimming trunks/swimsuit) beneath your wetsuit. Otherwise, when it comes to transition 1 (T1), you are risking serious embarrassment.

≡ Apply wetsuit lubricant to your neck, wrists, lower legs, ankles, feet, and wetsuit-leg bottoms before you put your wetsuit on. It will save you valuable seconds at T1 when you take it off.

≡ Put on your race swimming hat with plenty of time to spare, but leave your goggles dangling around your neck. Make sure you've applied any anti-fogging spray to your goggles before you get to the start line. Place the goggles over your eyes just before the starting gun goes off, so they don't mist up before you start swimming.

≡ Be one of the last to enter the water so that you can swim without being distracted by other competitors. At the back of the field you can avoid all the worst aspects of "the washing machine"—as the main swim pack is nicknamed (see page 118). You won't get accidentally kicked or punched, you'll avoid the worst of the churned-up water, no one will swim over the top of you, and you can follow the more experienced swimmers in front of you.

≡ If you breathe only on one side while you swim, choose a starting position on the opposite side of the main pack. That way, you can monitor other swimmers as you breathe.

≡ If you get nervous, distracted, or kicked during the swim, it's a good idea to stop, tread water, and compose yourself. Likewise, if your goggles mist up, there's nothing wrong with stopping to clear them.

Pro-Tip

Starting position for swim

Alistair Brownlee, Olympic triathlon gold medalist

"If it's one of your first races and you're not so confident, don't feel you need to start right in the middle. Instead start at the side or the back, where there are fewer people, until you get the confidence of being right in the middle of it. In any case, the time difference between the front and the back isn't that great."

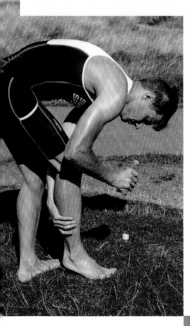

LUBRICATE YOUR WETSUIT

After your swim you need to strip quicker than a cheap lap-dancer, but getting a wetsuit off isn't always easy. To speed things up, it's advisable to apply a lubricant product. Smear it on your neck, wrists, feet, ankles, lower legs, and the bottom of your wetsuit legs. Be careful not to get it on your goggles—bring a towel so that you can wipe your hands.

Lubricant will also help prevent chafing, where the edge of the wetsuit rubs against your skin, and there's the added benefit that greased-up feet will slip into cycling shoes much more quickly at T1. But be warned: some petroleum jellies may damage your wetsuit, in which case triathlon-specific products such as Bodyglide will be much better. Check with the manufacturer first.

Pro-Tip

Removing a wetsuit

Steve Lumley, Malaysia-based triathlon coach

"Some elite triathletes can get a wetsuit off in six or eight seconds. Beginners tend to get flustered and waste a lot of time doing this. Using lubricant—and practicing taking off your wetsuit quickly—will save you loads of time."

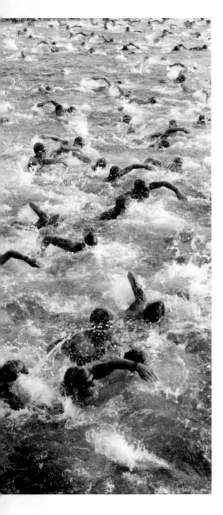

SWIMMING IN THE WASHING MACHINE

The start of the swim section is the part most beginners find the scariest: the thrashing of the water, the flailing of all those arms, the kicking of all those legs. The organized chaos of an open-water swim is often called "the washing machine." As a triathlon virgin, the most important thing is to try not to get flustered.

Start your swim section at the back or the edge of the field where you are unlikely to get accidentally punched or kicked by other swimmers. Bear in mind that when you're rounding a buoy there may well be a bottleneck of swimmers. You can avoid this by swimming in a wide arc around any buoys.

If you do find yourself troubled by other swimmers, you have two choices. You can either hold your swimming line and maintain your pace, knowing that less confident swimmers will move out of your way, or, alternatively, you can swim away from the washing machine to avoid any trouble. In this case you'll end up swimming a bit farther than the main pack of swimmers, but you'll exit the water a lot less stressed.

Open-water swimming shouldn't be a contact sport, but it often is. So be prepared for a little bit of argy-bargy in the water. If you find your goggles get accidentally dislodged by a fellow swimmer, don't panic, and don't stop swimming forward, otherwise other triathletes will start to swim over the top of you. Keep swimming forward, but move well away from the main pack, clear out your goggles, and then, once you've regained your confidence and composure, ease yourself back into the rhythm of the race.

Pro-Tip

The washing machine
Jonathan Brownlee, triathlon champion

"The swim section can be pretty chaotic. Remind yourself that when you're in a wetsuit you're absolutely fine. Don't worry. There's nothing that can go wrong; you're not going to drown because the buoyancy of the suit keeps you on top of the water. Practice swimming in your wetsuit in swimming pools before the race. Get your friends to rough you up a bit in the swimming pool so that you're used to the washing machine."

SIGHTING

To spare yourself from swimming farther than you need to, every few meters use a technique called sighting—that's where you use buoys in the water or landmarks on the shore to orient yourself in the right direction. (See sighting tips on page 44.)

In amateur triathlons, it's not unusual to see people swimming a long way off course before they realize they're going in the wrong direction. That's why you should try to sight every five or six strokes, if possible. Given enough time before the race, it's a great idea to practice on the actual swim course so that you can work out the best landmarks for sighting.

Never assume that the swimmers in front of you are swimming in the right direction. In the water, inexperienced triathletes are often like sheep, blindly following one another.

DRAFTING

Even basic drafting will save you valuable seconds and energy during the swim (see drafting tips, page 44), but you need to choose the right swimmer to draft behind. Don't draft behind someone who's slower than you because that will just slow you down. Equally, don't draft behind someone who's a lot faster than you, since you'll never keep up. The ideal is to find a swimmer who swims at the same speed or marginally faster than you. That way you'll either save energy or travel faster through the water. And be sure to adopt the optimal position when you draft: that's just behind the swimmer's feet (but not touching their feet) or to the side of their hip.

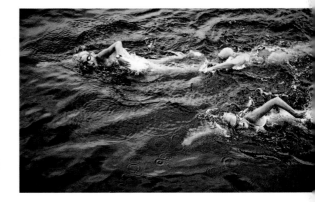

Drafting

Alistair Brownlee, Olympic triathlon gold medalist,

"You have to be swimming quite fast to make drafting worthwhile. If you're a beginner, and starting at the back, don't worry too much about drafting. If you're at the sharp end of the field, it definitely has an effect. Draft directly behind another swimmer to keep things simple. Drafting on the hip of a swimmer is quite difficult."

BUOY TURNS

On open-water swims, it can get quite congested at the buoys as swimmers make their turns. If you're a weaker swimmer, you may want to make wide turns around the buoys to avoid the inevitable melee. It will make your swim slightly longer, but a lot less stressful.

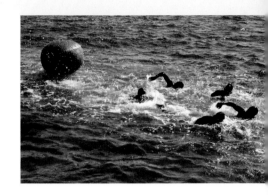

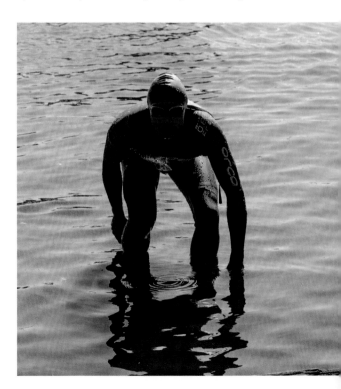

RACE STORIES

George Valentine, a 28-year-old blogger from Denver, USA, who took part in his first triathlon in 2011

"It was just a few minutes before the start of the race when I noticed my tires were soft. The gauge on my pump said they were at 90 psi. Another competitor told me, 'You need them up to at least 120 psi,' so I started pumping more. I got to 110 psi and suddenly the inner tube exploded. It sounded like a bomb had gone off. All the other competitors looked round and I felt like a right idiot. I didn't have a spare tube on me and I was really worried I wouldn't have time to buy one and fit it. Fortunately, the guy who had told me to get pumping lent me his spare inner tube, which I managed to fit with just a few minutes to spare before the start of the race. I ran and jumped into the water just as the starting klaxon went off."

EXITING THE WATER

On an open-water swim, keep swimming until the water is very shallow. Once it's around knee height, use your arms to push yourself to a standing position, raise your goggles onto your swimming cap, and then start jogging through the shallows. Once the water is shallow enough for there to be no risk of tripping over, you can start undoing your wetsuit. If you have extricated your torso and both arms by the time you reach dry land, you're doing well.

Removing your wetsuit quickly

Apply wetsuit lubricant before you put on your wetsuit (see page 117). Also, water acts as a lubricant, so with a bit of practice you should be able to whip off your wetsuit within a few seconds, provided you're still dripping wet from the swim.

1. On exiting the water, use one hand to undo the Velcro strap at the back of your neck and the other to gently pull down the zipper.

2. Release your left shoulder from the wetsuit and pull your left arm completely free.

3. Now use your left hand to release your right shoulder and pull your right arm completely free of the wetsuit.

4. Some triathletes completely remove their wetsuits immediately after exiting the water, since it's easier to remove a wetsuit when it's wet and it's quicker to run with the wetsuit over your shoulder.

But, if you prefer, you can always run to the transition area with your legs still in the wetsuit but the torso and arms dangling loose.

5. Once you're in the transition area, clutch the sides of the wetsuit and pull it as far down as you can over your waist and upper legs.

6. Stand on one side of the wetsuit and pull your leading leg free.

7. Stand on the other side of the wetsuit and pull your second leg free.

8. Leave your wetsuit, swimming hat, and goggles in your transition area.

Pro-Tip

Remove your wetsuit immediately

Mike Trees, ex-pro triathlete and multisport coach

"I always remove my wetsuit as soon as I can. Sometimes I start taking it off when I'm still in the water, hurdling over the waves. If you run to your bike in your wetsuit, the water will have dripped off the inside of it. It almost creates a vacuum between the suit and your skin, which makes it really difficult to get off."

T1 TRANSITION TIPS

Because of all the equipment needed, triathletes need to be meticulous about their transition area. On race day, don't leave any equipment at home. (See page 113 for an equipment checklist.)

There is usually a single transition area where you execute both T1 and T2. (Some have two separate areas, but to keep things simple we are assuming it's just the one transition area.)

1. Rack your bike in the correct bike rack, with the chain in an easy gear so you can pedal off quickly.

2. Hang your cycling helmet from the handlebars and hook your cycling glasses inside them.

3. If you're using clipless pedals, you may want to leave your cycling shoes clipped into your pedals to save time on T1. Many triathletes use elastic bands in order to keep their cycling shoes upright, even when they're running with the bike out of the transition area.

4. Next to your bike, lay a small towel down on the ground. This is where you're going to keep all your gear. The brighter the color of that towel, the better, since you'll then easily spot it from a distance as you enter the transition area.

5. Make sure the laces and tongues of your running shoes are loosened so you can get them on quickly. If you run in socks, place one sock in each shoe.

6. On your towel, place your race number and race belt, any cycling and running clothing, and your water bottle(s) and race food. Leave a small section of your towel clear so that you can wipe your feet on it when you arrive from the swim. After exiting the water, your wet feet will pick up all sorts of dirt—not what you need inside your cycling shoes.

7. Remember that you risk a time penalty or disqualification if you exit the transition area without your helmet on and secure. For this reason, many triathletes get into the habit of putting their helmet on in T1 before they touch any other equipment.

8. Most triathletes cycle and run in the clothing they wear beneath their wetsuit (i.e. a tri suit or swimming trunks/swimsuit). But if you're more comfortable changing into cycling shorts and cycling jersey for the bike section, then go ahead. It will cost more time, and might involve having to get changed with a towel wrapped round your body—not always so graceful.

9. Remember to clip on your number belt and race number.

10. Remove your bike from its rack and wheel it as you run to the end of the transition area. Some triathletes can wheel their bike using only the saddle to guide it. Others need to hold the saddle and the handlebars to guide it. The latter technique means you need to be careful not to trip over your pedals.

`Pro-Tip`

Socks

Rob Griffiths, head of TrainingBible Coaching UK

"You might want to wear a pair of thin running socks for both the bike and run sections of triathlon. When you become more experienced in the sport you can get away without socks altogether. If you're racing early in the season, you can get really cold feet. Coming straight out of the pool, they may be freezing when you first get on the bike. If you suffer from poor circulation, it may be better all round to lose 20 seconds in T1 putting on your socks. At the start of the run, some triathletes get that bizarre sensation where it feels like they have no feet. It's almost like you're running on the stubs of your legs, but that feeling will normally pass after the first mile or so."

RACE STORIES

Nick Hutchings, a 37-year-old producer from Oxfordshire, UK, who took part in his second London Triathlon in 2012

"It was just 20 minutes before the start of the race and I was doing a last-minute check through all my gear when I realized I had my wetsuit but no tri suit. I actually owned four of them, but I'd left them all at home. So I started panicking, running up and down the bike rack area like a headless chicken. What was I going to do? I couldn't very well finish the swim section and then cycle and run in my wetsuit. I certainly couldn't compete in the nude. It quickly dawned on me that I'd done two months of hard training and it was all for nothing.

"I ended up rushing to one of the stalls in the competitors' village and buying the first tri suit I could find. It was double the market price, it didn't fit properly, and the padding was hanging down well below my groin. But I didn't have any choice. I made it to the start line just in time. During the bike section my low-grade tri suit gave me horrendous bum burn; during the run it was bleeding nipples. Not much fun."

BIKE MOUNTING

There are several ways to mount a bike while on the run—from the left, from the right, leading leg first, leading leg second, but it's a technique you need to practice if you want to save time. The easiest method involves placing your outside leg onto the pedal nearest you first before swinging your inside leg over the saddle onto the second pedal. Your method should vary, depending on whether you're cycling in trainers, in cycling shoes, with flat pedals, or with clipless pedals.

If you're using clipless pedals and your cycling shoes are already clipped into your pedals, you need to get your feet inside the shoes as quickly as possible. Start by placing just your left toes into your left shoe, with your right foot resting on top of your right shoe. Wiggle your left toes so that all of your left foot except the heel is inside the shoe. Now reach down and slip the heel of your shoe over your left heel. Tighten the shoe strap. Now apply the same process to your right foot. It sounds complicated but, with a bit of practice, you'll soon have it down to a fine art.

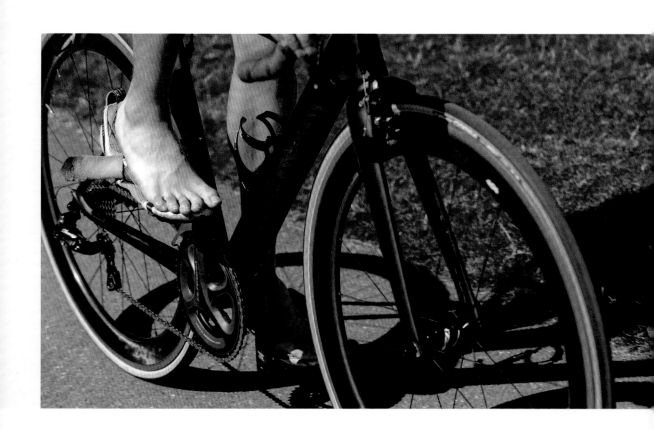

BIKE RACING TIPS

It's during the bike section that you'll have the best opportunity to drink and eat. During the swim it's too early in the race and you'll be too wet. And during the run you'll be jogging up and down too much to ingest food unless you've stopped at a feeding station. That's why the bike ride is food and drink time. But wait until you've established a rhythm on your bike before you start eating.

It's rare that you'll need to eat on a Sprint-distance triathlon. On Olympic distances, however, you should try to consume a few carbohydrates during the bike section. Perhaps keep a couple of energy bars in the back pocket of your tri suit, or taped to your handlebars. There should be at least one full bottle of your chosen drink in a bottle cage on your bike.

ENERGY DRINKS AND GELS

Many triathlon races offer free energy drinks and energy gels to the competitors at feeding stations. When it comes to ingredients and taste, different brands vary enormously. Many of them contain huge amounts of sugar. It's a good idea to bring your own food to races so that you consume the type of food, or brand of food, that your body is used to. When you're training, you can learn what amounts and what types of food your body ideally needs. That way, come race day, your stomach won't have any nasty surprises.

Pro-Tip

Race Nutrition

Jonathan Brownlee, triathlon champion

"On an Olympic-distance triathlon you only need to eat on the bike section. I take an energy gel after 20km and 35km of the bike section. Sip an energy drink all the way through the bike section, too. Then you'll be fine for the run."

🏁 RACE STORIES

Paul Parrish, a 49-year-old marketing director, who in 2014 took part in one of the toughest triathlons on the planet: the Enduroman Arch to Arc, a 290-mile punishment that requires running from London to Dover, swimming the English Channel, and cycling from Calais to Paris.

"During the swim we hit heavy weather after six hours. When I wasn't near the coast in the time I had mentally thought I would be, I thought I had blown the whole attempt. To carry on swimming when you believe all hope is gone is incredibly hard when you are completely spent. It was tough and gruesome. The muscles in the left side of my back seized up for the last hour and a half of the swim, and that affected my stroke badly. But I was beyond caring about the physical at that point. All the pain was in my head. It was a very lonely place to be."

Finally, after 17.5 hours in the water, 10 of them in complete darkness, Paul felt his hands strike the sand of the French coast. "I sobbed with joy all the way up the beach," he says. He reached Paris in a total of 84 hours and 44 minutes.

DON'T DRAFT

Remember that drafting is forbidden in most triathlon races. Race rules demand a minimum gap between bikes. Unless you're a very confident cyclist, you won't want to ride too close to the riders in front of you anyway for fear of clipping their back wheel with your front wheel.

HILLS AND CORNERING

At beginner-level triathlons, you can win valuable time on uphill sections and corners. (See page 64 for hill climbing and cornering tips.)

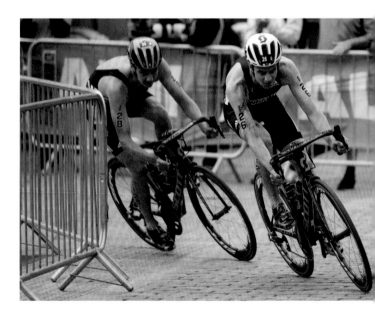

RACE AT YOUR OWN PACE

On your first triathlon you'll be tempted to speed through the bike section. Remember to race at your own pace. Don't be egged on too much by the other competitors. Go too fast on the bike and you'll have little energy left for the run.

T2 TRANSITION TIPS

If you're clipped into clipless pedals, it's likely you're wearing a pair of cycling shoes that are very tricky to run in. If that's the case, you'll need to extricate your feet well in advance of the end of the bike ride so you can run through the T2 transition in bare feet.

QUICK BIKE DISMOUNT

Just like in the Wild West, a quick dismount can make all the difference between glory and ignominy. If you're using normal flat pedals, it's a lot easier.

At the end of the bike section, around 10 meters before you reach the dismount line, flip one leg over the back wheel so that you're freewheeling along with just one foot on the pedal. Then slow the bike down and, before you pass the dismount line, step forward with your rear leg and start running alongside the bike. You'll find this is so much quicker than bringing the bike to a halt before dismounting, since then you'd have to start running again from a standstill.

If you're wearing clipless pedals, you need to extricate your feet from your cycling shoes well before the dismount line. To do this, just before the end of the bike section, while you're still cycling, you stop pedaling and allow the bike to freewheel along. Then you bend down, loosen the Velcro straps on your shoes, slip your feet out, and place them on top of the shoes (which will still be clipped into the cleats). Now you can continue

pedaling, but with your feet completely out of your shoes.

When you eventually dismount (see below), you can then run across the transition area in your socks or bare feet.

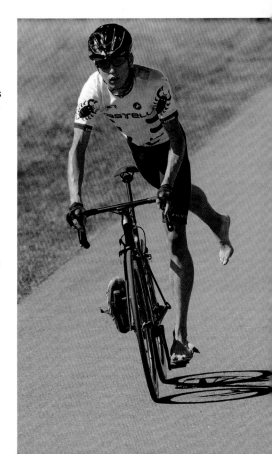

HELMET FASTENING

Triathlon race organizers are super strict about helmet wear during the bike section, insisting that you keep your skid lid on until you've racked your bike. Many a triathlete has fallen foul of this helmet rule. Even experienced racers occasionally get penalized at T2 for removing their helmet too early. Get into the habit of keeping your helmet on even until after you've put on your running shoes. Some helmet clips and straps get twisted up after you've been using them a while. It's well worth making sure yours is adjusted, and functioning properly, before the race.

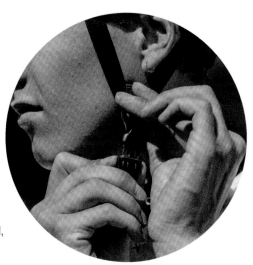

ELASTIC LACES

Elastic laces are pulled tight rather than tied like normal laces. There are several different styles on the market. Most can be fitted to most normal running shoes, in place of the existing laces, essentially turning lace-ups into slip-ons. You won't need them for training but during the race they will save you valuable seconds at the T2 transition. There's also no risk that your laces might come undone in the middle of your run section.

Like all equipment, practice using elastic laces well before race day. Some triathletes prefer to sit down when putting on running shoes, while others prefer to stand. Don't fit them too tightly. Make sure the tension is correct. Too loose and your shoes could fly off, too tight and they could be very uncomfortable.

RUNNING RACE TIPS

Be prepared for heavy legs as you switch from cycling to running. There will be a strange sensation in your lower legs as your muscles adapt. It can be very discomfiting, especially for debutant triathletes, but the feeling will normally pass after a few hundred meters.

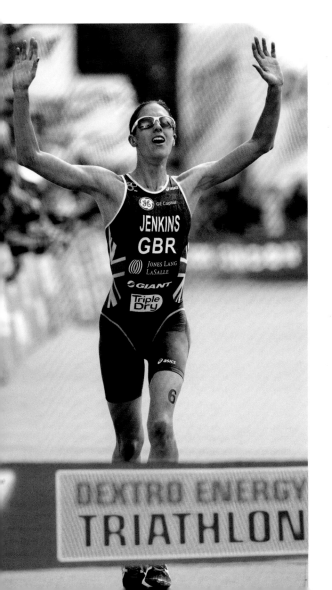

FINISH LINE

Enjoy your moment of glory as you cross the finish line. A lot of triathletes obsess about stopping their stopwatch at the exact moment they cross the line, but this means you'll be looking downward when the race photographer takes your photo. Forget your stopwatch—after all, the race officials are recording your time for you. Instead, look up toward the photographer and smile. Who knows? You may even get your mugshot in the local media?

Pro-Tip

Feeding stations
Alistair Brownlee, Olympic triathlon gold medalist

"If you're doing Olympic distance, don't feel you have to stop at feeding stations during the run. If it's hot, you might just grab some water; sip it or pour it over your head."

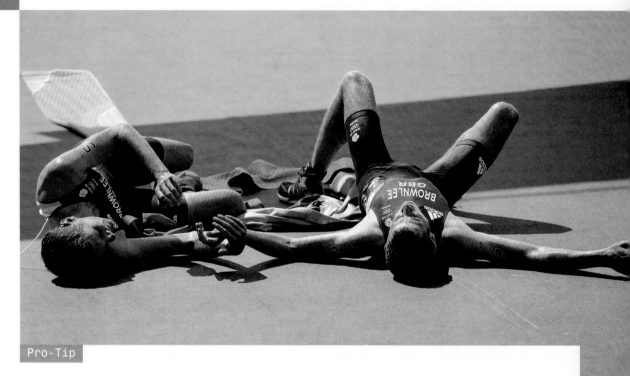

Break up the distances

Luke Tyburski, who completed a 2,000-km triathlon challenge from Morocco to Monaco in 12 days

"I use what I call 'the rule of five.' I break up every long section into five smaller sections. And I find this works, whatever the distance. So, for example, in the Olympic-distance triathlon, you could break the 1,500m swim into five 300m swims. Or you could break up the 40-km bike section into five 8-km rides. It makes it much more manageable.

"With the first of the five sections, you simply tell yourself, 'Right, this is the first one. I just have to get it done.' When it comes to the second one, you know what it's going to be like, and you know you're going to be hurting, so there are no surprises. The third section is the most difficult. This is the top of the mountain. This is where you really challenge yourself. With the fourth one, you have to think to yourself, after this I've only got one more to go. Finally, the fifth one is the last one so, mentally, it's easy. Job done."

TRIATHLON LEGENDS
Emma Snowsill (Australia)

BORN: June 15, 1981, Gold Coast, Australia
OLYMPIC GAMES GOLD MEDAL: Beijing 2008
ITU WORLD CHAMPION: 2003, 2005, 2006

Back in 2002, after her boyfriend was killed by the driver of a stolen car, Snowsill suffered depression and very nearly abandoned triathlon altogether. Fortunately, her boyfriend's sister persuaded her to start training again. In the years that followed she saw glory at the Olympic Games, the Commonwealth Games, and in the ITU World Championships.

After she picked up an illness while on holiday in Bali, recurring problems with her body's immune system forced Snowsill to retire from triathlon in 2014 at the age of 33.

She is married to the other Beijing Olympics triathlon gold medalist Jan Frodeno (see page 55).

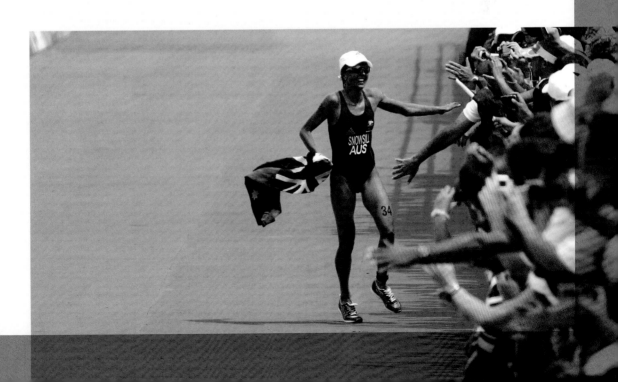

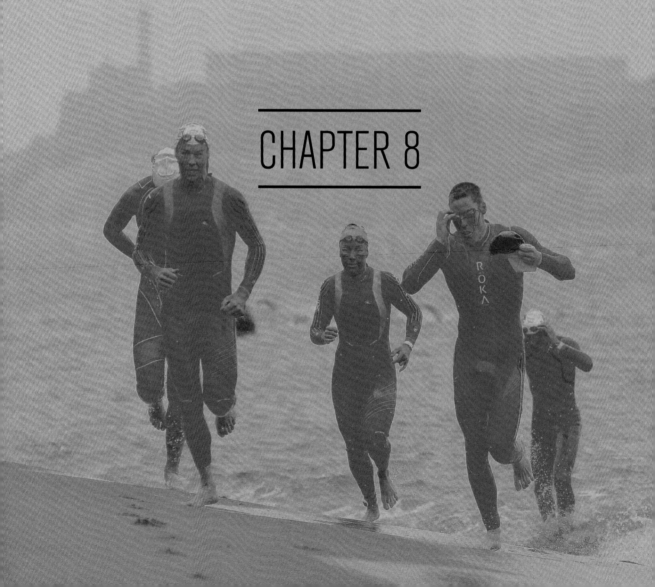

CHAPTER 8

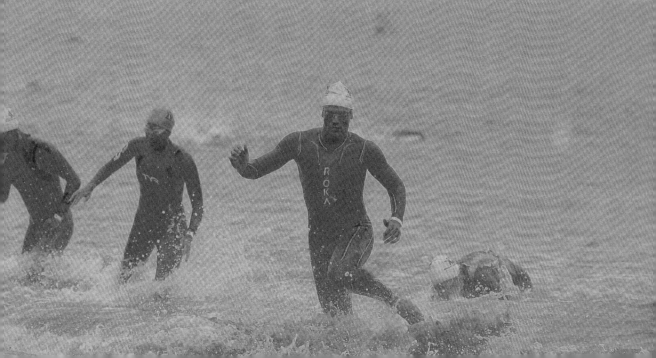

THE WORLD'S GREATEST TRIATHLONS

NEED A NEW CHALLENGE AFTER COMPLETING THE OLYMPIC DISTANCE?

On any weekend of the year, somewhere on this huge planet of ours, athletes are taking part in a triathlon. Some of these races are tiny affairs with just a handful of competitors, egged on by their loved ones. Others are enormous international events, with hundreds of athletes, thousands of spectators, full-time staff, and wall-to-wall media coverage, so that they have almost come to define the countryside through which their routes wind.

Here we pay tribute to some of the world's most important triathlons; the ones that should be on every seasoned triathlete's bucket list.

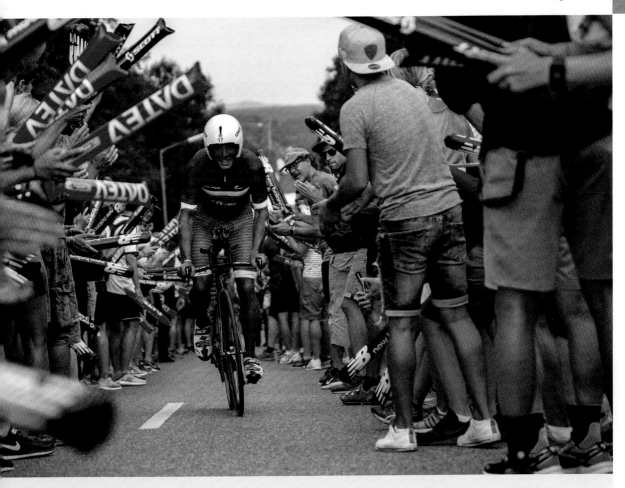

CHALLENGE ROTH

Roth, Germany

It may be the same length as an Ironman, but there's plenty going on to distract the weary participants in this German triathlon. Perhaps too much. After all, there are normally well over 3,000 individuals and around 650 relay teams taking part, all cheered on by over a quarter of a million beery spectators. The organizers claim it is "the world's biggest long-distance triathlon."

After a good two days of pre-race festivities, including the obligatory sporting of traditional dirndl dresses and lederhosen, the event kicks off with a 3.8km swim in one of Roth's major water courses, the Main-Donau-Kanal. This is followed by a 180-km bike leg, much of which is enlivened by huge throngs of Teutonically keen supporters wielding rattles, cowbells, and mugs of beer, all shouting and singing at the top of their voices. Close your eyes and you'll think you're at a Bundesliga soccer match or in a beer hall during Oktoberfest.

The marathon-distance run reaches its climax in the Roth triathlon stadium which, once the final competitor crosses the line, is lit up with a huge fireworks display and more reveling. That's enough to flush out even the most stubborn lactic acid.

ESCAPE FROM ALCATRAZ

San Francisco, California, USA

Prisons are always resoundingly grim places. But Alcatraz Federal Penitentiary, a high-security island lockup in the middle of San Francisco Bay, was perhaps grimmer than most. This was where Al Capone, George "Machine Gun" Kelly, Alvin "Creepy" Karpis, and various other reprobates passed many years at the government's leisure.

It's also the starting point for a famous triathlon called Escape from Alcatraz. Although the course of the race has changed over the years, a recent edition saw athletes starting by diving off a boat moored just off Alcatraz Island, and swimming 1.5 miles across the bay. "A 7:30am plunge from the San Francisco Belle into the icy cold water," is how organizers entice new participants.

Then follows an 18-mile bike leg that takes in city sights such as the Presidio, Camino del Mar,

the Palace of the Legion of Honor, and Golden Gate Park. After that, the 8-mile run hugs much of the coastline and includes a section beneath the famous Golden Gate Bridge. But the most grueling bit of all is the 400-step climb up the Equinox Sand Ladder, with uneven log steps and a hand cable to pull on. "This experience will drain the legs of even the best professionals," the organizers add. "The stairs are to the run what the currents and waves are to the swim."

In the 1979 movie *Escape from Alcatraz*, starring Clint Eastwood, the prison warden famously boasts: "Since I've been warden, a few people have tried to escape. Most of them have been recaptured. Those that haven't have been killed or drowned in the bay. No one has ever escaped from Alcatraz. And no one ever will!"

Be warned.

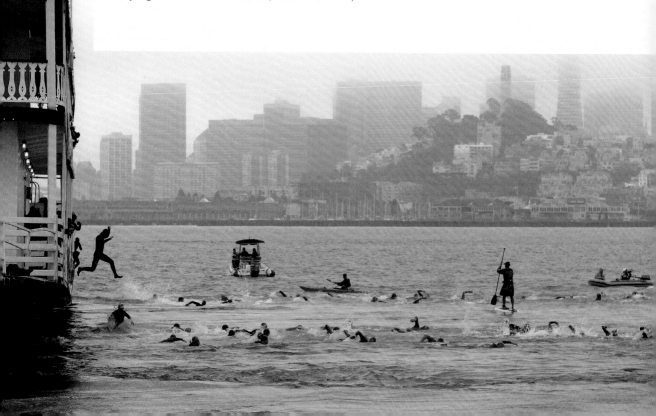

XTERRA WORLD CHAMPIONSHIPS

Maui, Hawaii, USA

Once you exit the swim, the vast majority of triathlons stage the bike and the run sections on tarmac. Not Xterra, however. This global series of races—culminating in the annual Xterra World Championships, on the Hawaiian island of Maui—is strictly off-road. So where you'd usually race with a road bike or tri bike, you need a mountain bike, and where you'd usually run on the road, you run on dirt trails instead.

The course of the world championships has changed many times since it was first set in 1996, but the latest version saw athletes negotiating a "rough-water swim" of just under a mile, a 20-mile bike ride with 2,800 ft of climbing that loops the lower slopes of the West Maui Mountains, and a 6.5-mile run that takes in dirt trails, oleander forests, a mountain lake at 700 ft above sea level, steep downhills and a sandy beach.

"It's an honest endurance challenge, that's for sure," says race director "Kahuna Dave" Nicholas. "This course is not just for survivors, but for those with the skills and endurance to ride the bike well and fast, and still have enough left in their legs to climb some more; and, more importantly, descend some steep downhills on a really challenging trail run. The scenery is something that not many people get a chance to see."

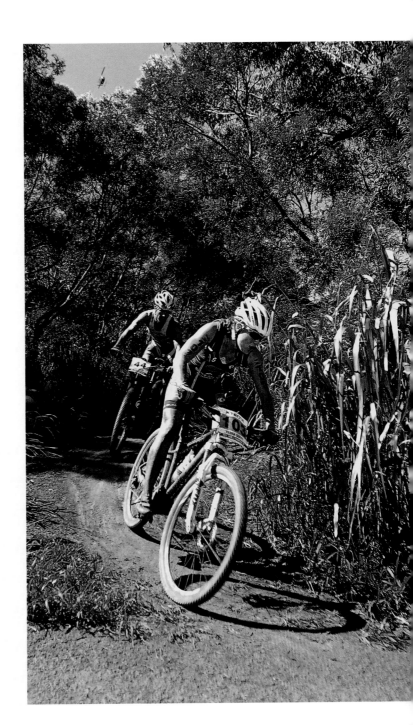

NORSEMAN XTREME TRIATHLON

Eidfjord, Norway

The Norwegians are a hardy lot. When it comes to sport, many of them adopt a hard-man attitude that they must have inherited from their Viking ancestors. That Viking spirit is very much alive during the Norseman Xtreme Triathlon, a long-distance race staged in a beautifully rugged region of southern Norway.

It all kicks off with a 4-m dive off a ferry into the cold waters of the Hardangerfjord, followed by a 3.8km swim. Then there's a 180-km bike ride and a marathon-distance run across the Hardangervidda mountains. The total ascent of the race is 5,000m, ending with a steep climb to the rocky summit of Mount Gaustatoppen, 1,850m above sea level, where weather conditions are often very harsh. "The weather can be anything from brilliantly beautiful to blasting blizzard, sometimes all in one day," warn the organizers. "You get the sense of being marooned in a vast landscape only suited for reindeer and hard rocks where there's no one to see you, hear you, or cheer you on. It's just you, your bike, and the will to make it to the finish line."

Oh, and a note about the locals. "Please be friendly to the locals," the organizers request. "They are totally amazed that you came, and they think you're completely nuts to be doing this. You are."

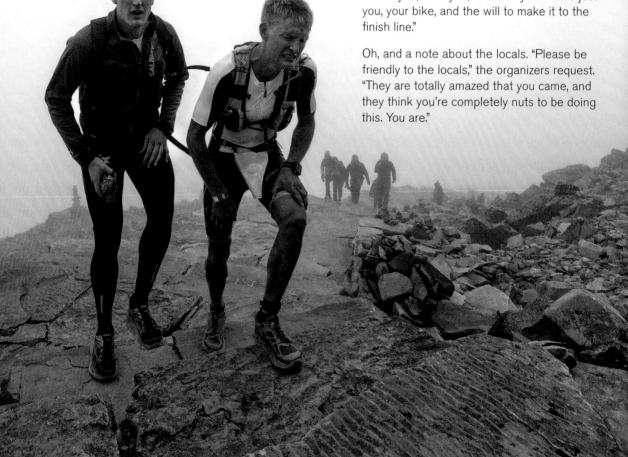

CHALLENGE WANAKA

Lake Wanaka, New Zealand

A beach start, a swim through warm water so clean you can drink it, followed by bike and run legs across mountainous national parks, and alongside lakes and rivers… this Ironman-distance triathlon is regularly voted one of the world's most scenic. Indeed, there's certainly lots of eye candy to keep competitors distracted as they negotiate the beautiful nature of Lake Wanaka and its surrounding areas. No wonder around 1,600 of them turn up to this event in New Zealand's South Island every year to take part. The post-race party atmosphere is great, too, with music and fireworks carrying on until the last athlete crosses the finish line.

"Challenge Wanaka is such a buzz, and an amazing course and atmosphere," says top New Zealand triathlete and 2014 runner-up Richard Ussher. "At Wanaka you will feel the real challenge of all the elements: sun, heat, wind, hills, and off-road running," adds Canadian competitor Luke Dragstra.

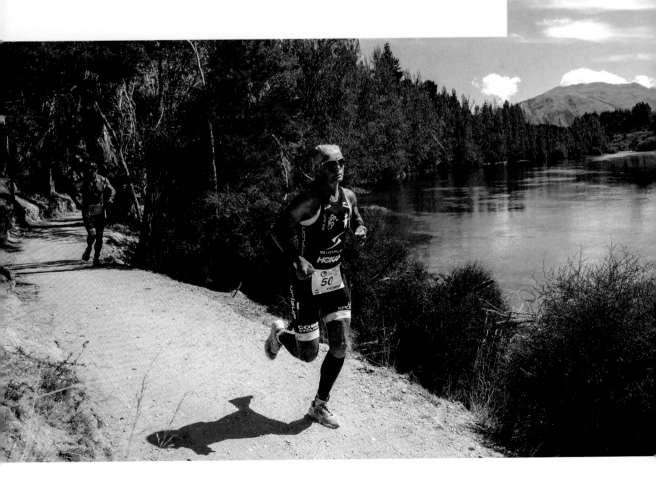

LONDON TRIATHLON

London, UK

The London Triathlon certainly isn't the toughest triathlon out there since it's very flat and features distances ranging from Super Sprint (400m swim, 10km bike, 2.5km run) up to Olympic Plus (1,500m swim, 80km bike, 10km run). But it's a classic in that it claims to be "the largest triathlon in the world," with more than 13,000 athletes and 30,000 spectators. Choose the longer route and it also takes in some pretty special London sights, including Big Ben, the London Eye, Tower Bridge, the Tower of London, the O2, Canary Wharf, and a long stretch of the River Thames. It's open to all standards of triathlete, from complete beginners to elite standard.

Proceedings kick off in one of the UK's largest exhibition centers, ExCeL, in east London. From here competitors swim in the water of Docklands before embarking on a very flat bike route, and then a very flat run. As well as the famous London landmarks, what really drives competitors on is the constant cheering of the thousands of fans lining the route. Just like the city that hosts it, there's never a quiet moment in this race.

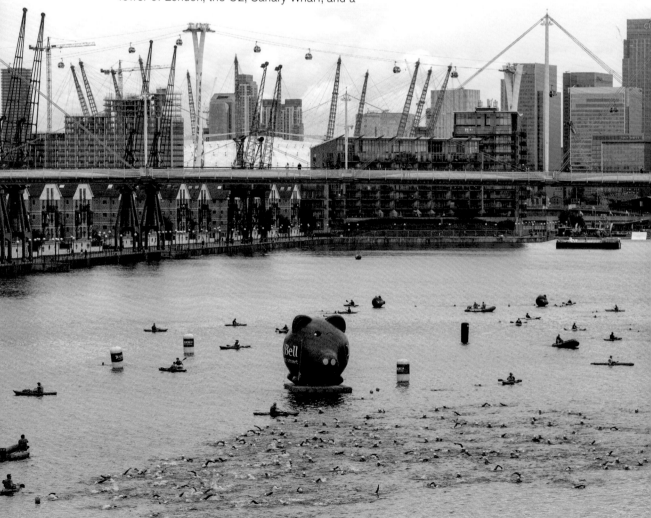

ENDUROMAN ARCH TO ARC TRIATHLON

London, UK, to Paris, France

London has its famous Marble Arch. Paris has its even more famous Arc de Triomphe. The two landmarks are 213 miles (343km) apart as the crow flies, with lots of countryside and, of course, the English Channel in between them. Surely it's not possible to race from one to the other, by running, cycling, and swimming?

Au contraire. Truly intrepid athletes take part in a race called the Enduroman Arch to Arc triathlon. It must be one of the longest and most daunting point-to-point triathlons on the planet.

The odyssey starts with an 87-mile (140-km) run from central London's Marble Arch to Dover, on the Kent coast. Then comes the toughest bit— the swim across the English Channel from England to France (at least 21 miles or 34km, depending on sea currents). Finally, there's the 181-mile (290-km) bike ride to Paris.

Only a few dozen athletes have ever completed the challenge. Frenchman Cyril Blanchard, a member of Beauvais triathlon club in northern France, set a new record in 2016. He ran London to Dover in 18 hours, 35 minutes. His cross-Channel swim took 14 hours, 47 minutes. And his bike ride to Paris was completed in 13 hours, 48 minutes. Factor in the obligatory waits at the transitions and you get an overall time of 59 hours and 56 minutes. Not as fast as Eurostar but impressive all the same.

"It's over! It was very, very, very, very tough," he said, raising his bike above his head in a victory salute at the Arc de Triomphe. "Victorious!" he added with a whoop of delight.

Blanchard had trained for up to 20 hours a week in the run-up to his mighty triathlon. "This is a full-on sport which is mostly about mental strength," he explained. "Even with loads of training, the power of a triathlete is his mind."

In 2017, tragically, a triathlete called Douglas Waymark died while competing in the event.

IRONMAN WORLD CHAMPIONSHIP

Big Island, Hawaii, USA

Thanks to a history dating back to the late 1970s, and some brilliant marketing, the Ironman triathlon series is arguably the most famous in the world. Consisting of a 2.4-mile swim, a 112-mile bike ride, and a standard-distance marathon, the races have gradually spread all over the globe so that now there are over 40 events across six continents (plus another 100 or so half Ironman events), culminating in Hawaii's annual Ironman World Championship.

This season finale amalgamates around 2,000 athletes who have accrued enough points from Ironman events elsewhere during the same season. There are therefore no stragglers.

With more than a little hyperbole, the race organizers explain the motivation behind the triathletes who make it to the start line. "Those who come here, they want the journey to mean something; for their efforts to change who they are, and who they will become. While they come from different countries, different backgrounds, they share a common calling. For them, life is not meant to be seen, it is meant to be lived. So they rise up and then they raise the bar and push again. Blood, sweat, and tears connected to their very souls. These are the athletes of Ironman who continue to pursue something more; who, no matter what, believe that anything is possible."

On completing a normal Ironman race, many athletes mark their achievement with an Ironman logo tattoo on their calf. Should they cross the finish line of the Ironman World Championship, this tattoo ought to be obligatory.

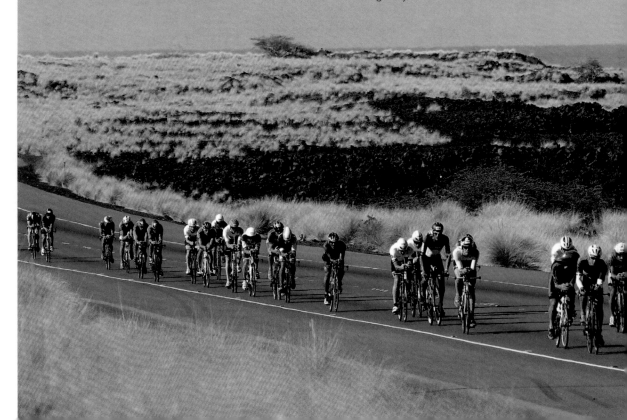

ULTRAMAN WORLD CHAMPIONSHIPS

Big Island, Hawaii, USA

"An athletic odyssey of personal rediscovery." That's how the Ultraman World Championships—one of the world's most testing triathlons—is sold. And you'd better believe it. This legendary Hawaii sports event is so long it can break the very fittest triathletes.

There are a total of 320 miles to cover: first the 6.2-mile open-ocean swim in the sea off Hawaii's Big island; then a 261-mile bike ride on the island's roads; finally a 52-mile road run. The event is staged over three days but with cut-off times imposed on each stage to eliminate any stragglers.

Each section offers its own interesting challenges. The swim is especially testing, with triathletes facing brushes with jellyfish or Portuguese man o' war—"whose stings may cause severe discomfort," warn the organizers rather coolly. For that reason, wetsuits are recommended. Ocean swells can be strong, throwing the swimmers about like corks in bottles. And there are risks of laceration from sharp outcrops of lava and coral, or spiky sea urchins. "Since stepping on one of these may cause painful and bothersome injury that may even prevent further participation, caution should be exercised when in shallow water," the organizers advise of the latter.

But there are plenty of other tests in store, in both the bike and the run sections, as the following competitors recount. "I felt very sick and nauseous," said Jack Nosco of his bike ordeal. "I threw up several times and was forced to get off and walk—a first for me ever to have had to walk my bike. My wife did a wonderful job in convincing me to continue."

2000 competitor John Girmsey rested for two hours after exiting the swim but still got into trouble at the start of the bike ride. "The initial long climb took its toll and my legs were cramping," he said. "I started sucking down a lot of salt packets after that to stop the cramps but it took several hours before I had them under control again." On the run section he placed bags of ice under his hat to keep cool. "It proved to be a lifesaver."

1998 competitor Rick Kent found the weather unforgiving on the downhill sections of his bike ride. "It was hairy as hell coming down," he recalled. "I'm normally pretty fearless in these situations but sanity ruled it out. The rain and wind, along with the severe drop in temperature, made it hard to even ride. I was shaking really badly. All I had on was a sleeveless jersey and shorts. I couldn't even change my hand position to brake."

After winning the 1995 Ultraman, Kevin Cutjar described his ordeal as "much more than a long-distance race. It's a journey! I feel honored to have been amongst the few who have experienced what has been called one of the most demanding physical challenges ever devised by man."

INDEX

Allen, Mark 45
arm movement, running 82
athletics tracks 76

Badmann, Natascha 61
bikes 48–54
  bike fit 52, 53, 54
  frame size 51
  handling skills 62–63
  hybrid/street bikes 49
  mountain bikes 49, 51
  mounting/dismounting on
    the run 124, 127
  parts of a bike 52–53
  repairs 58–60
  road bikes/racing bikes 49, 51
  securing 89
  tri bars 49, 53, 54, 67
  tri bikes 49, 50
  turbo trainers 68
bras, sports 80
breathing, bilateral 36, 44
brick workouts 87–88, 89
Brownlee, Alistair 35, 114, 117,
  119, 129
Brownlee, Jonathan 15, 35, 50,
  118, 125
buoy turns 120

cadence
  cycling 63
  running 82
Challenge Roth 135
Challenge Wanaka 139
clipless pedals 53, 122, 124,
  127
clothing
  cycling 56
  running 77, 79–80
  swimming 31–34
compression clothing 80
cooling down 22
cornering 64, 126
cramps 89
cycling
  brick workouts 88, 89
  drills 65–68
  race day 122–128
  training 46–71
  see also bikes

delayed onset muscle soreness
  (DOMS) 17
drafting
  cycling 67, 126
  swimming 42, 44, 119
drag 38, 43

endurance training 66
Enduroman Arch to Arc 126,
  141
energy drinks and gels 21, 125
equipment 14
  cycling 48–57
  running 77–80
  swimming 31–34
Escape from Alcatraz 136
eyewear
  cycling 56
  swimming 34, 116

feeding stations 129
finish line 129
fitness 13
foot strike 78, 81
Frodeno, Jan 55, 131
front crawl 37–38

gear changing 63
gloves, cycling 57
goals 22, 23, 24
goggles 34, 116
Gomez, Javier 71
gyms 15, 75

Half Ironman 12
hats 80
helmets 57, 128
hills
  cycling 64, 66, 126
  running 83
history of the triathlon 7–8
hydration 21, 114

International Triathlon Union
  (ITU) 8
interval training
  cycling 66
  running 83
Ironman 8, 12
  World Championship 45, 55,
    61, 71, 115, 142

jackets 79
Johnstone, Jack 7

knee lift, running 82

leggings 79
London Triathlon 140
long-distance runs 83

Mission Bay Triathlon 7
Moss, Julie 45
motivation 17, 23, 25, 70

newbies 9, 12–13
Newby-Fraser, Paula 115
Norseman Xtreme Triathlon 138
number belt 57, 123
nutrition 20–21, 112
  race day 114, 125, 129

Olympic Games 8, 35, 55, 131
Olympic (standard) 12, 19
  training plan 102–109
open water swimming 30,
  43–44

park running 76
pedaling 62
popularity of triathlons 8–9, 15
posture, running 81

race day 110–130
  cycling 122–128
  kit preparation 113
  morning of the race 114
  night before 112
  pre-race food 114
  running 129
  swimming 116–121
  transition stages 122–123,
    127–128
race distances 12
race rules 112
recovery 22
rest days 17, 93
road running 75
running
  athletics tracks 76
  brick workouts 87–88, 89
  clothes and equipment 77–80
  drills 83
  long-distance runs 83
  park running 76
  race day 129
  road running 75
  techniques 81–82
  training 72–83
  treadmills 75
  woodland trails and
    countryside 76

safety 30, 43, 57
shoes
  cycling 122, 124, 127
  elastic laces 128
  running 77–78, 122
shorts 79
sighting 44, 119
Snowsill, Emma 55, 131
socks 79, 123
Sprint 13, 19, 48
  distance 12
  training plan 94–101

swim hats 34, 116
swimming
  brick workouts 87–88, 89
  drills 41–42
  equipment and wetsuits 31–34
  open water swimming 30,
    43–44
  pools 28–29
  race day 116–121
  techniques 36–40
  training 26–45
  training aids 34
  "washing machine" 116, 118

T-shirts 80
time penalties 122
timing chip 113
touch turns 38–39
training 15–19, 25
  apps and journal 17
  cycling 46–71
  group training 17, 25, 67
  overtraining 16–17
  running 72–83
  swimming 26–45
  tapering 19
  transition training 16, 84–90
training schedules 90–109
  Olympic 102–109
  Sprint 94–101
transition stages 13, 122–123,
  127–128
  components 87
transition training 16, 84–89
tri suits 33, 116
tumble turns 40
turbo trainers 68
Tyburski, Luke 70, 130

Ultraman World Championship
  143

warming up 65, 114
"washing machine" 116, 118
wetsuits 31–32
  lubricant 31–32, 116, 117
  putting on/removal 32, 44,
    117, 120–121

XTERRA World Championship
  71, 137